MW01385493

BRADBURY MUSCLE COURSE

BRADBURY MUSCLE COURSE

A no-nonsense approach for achieving a lean and muscular physique

Beau Bradbury

Copyright © Beau Bradbury

All rights reserved. No part of this book may be reproduced or transmitted in any form or by any means without the written permission from the author. All trademarks are the exclusive property of the author.

ISBN-13: 9781539121466
ISBN-10: 1539121461

Disclaimer:

All inherent forms of exercise involve potential risks. The author and publisher advise readers to take full responsibility for their safety and know their limits. Before embarking on the following suggestions and training program obtain a licensed physician's prior approval. Inspect your equipment to make sure that it is well maintained and fit for use. Never take any risks beyond your level of experience, aptitude, fitness and training. The author and publisher are not responsible in any way for any adverse effects or any injury resulting from the use of the information presented. The training and dietary guidelines in this book are not intended to replace any exercise and dietary program prescribed by your doctor.

Dedication

This book is dedicated to all of the people who desperately wanted to change their body for the better, but struggled to find out how. This book is your solution.

Godspeed my friend.

Table of Contents

Part 1: Why the *Bradbury Muscle Course?*

1

It's All About Muscle

The only way to kick off this book is to talk about what we are all here for: MUSCLE! In a time when many people are fooled by tricky and misleading marketers, it is hard to find something that is truly honest nowadays. Many times potential solutions are presented in such a way that the only thing holding you back is the money in your pocket. Money that can buy their miracle powder or special machine. The glaring problem is that, more often than not, these outlandish claims never live up to the hype and simply do not work! Not only have I personally fallen for these lies in the past, but millions of others have too. The truth is, the fitness industry is BIG BUSINESS. Unfortunately, any big business will attract plenty of hucksters. These high mach personalities live by the motto of do whatever it takes to get ahead. Many times this means professionally executed attacks of deceit, trickery, and empty promises. These heartless swindlers care about one thing and one thing only…YOUR MONEY. To get it they will go at great lengths of using deception and create mass confusion amongst the poor misguided souls that are in their crosshairs. They aim to sell you over-hyped promises and the delusion of easy and fast success. The truth is that no quick fixes actually work. The trouble is it simply does not work that way and your "promised" results go fleeing away once again. This is why I love muscle. Muscle cannot lie. Muscle is honest. It's been said that a great physique will earn you respect in an instant. This is because you cannot buy one. You cannot inherit one. You cannot fake a great physique. You cannot steal one. You cannot copy one. Most importantly, you cannot lie about having one. Looks don't lie and if you've earned a superb physique people will know within a nanosecond without you having to say a single word. Muscle is one thing that is truly honest! Frankly, you either have it or you don't. Like a bright star shining in the dark night, muscle is only EARNED through dedication, discipline and hard work. It can vanish rather quickly if not carefully maintained. Subconsciously, people will instantly have respect and admiration for you when they see you've put in the work required and earned yourself a stellar physique. Only the insecure will make weak, snickering comments to their friends. They will say things like "I think he is on the juice" or the common "I don't want to ever look like that." In wimpy and futile efforts they try to belittle your obvious accomplishment. This is a failing attempt to try to protect their fragile ego and mask their obvious insecurities. Mark my words. THIS WILL HAPPEN TO YOU! Take these attacks as a compliment, because if they ain't talking about you, it means you ain't doing anything. Never take it personally, because these jokers can't face the fact that you've done the hard work required and they simply have not. Jealousy is always a bad perfume. These people, either out of sheer laziness or a lack of ambition, have not earned what you've earned. Therefore, they try to belittle the importance of a commanding physique although their audience is usually none or small at best. You on the other hand will have done the program, pushed through the tough reps and will acquire the undeniable symbol of power and discipline. You will start to reap all kinds of rewards. Doors, once closed, will start to open up for you. People will treat you differently than before. Opportunities are abound for the few who have traveled the treacherous roads of endless sets and reps with heavy iron. Most importantly, you will learn self respect, discipline and sacrifice. Your confidence will soar. By sowing the seed of hard work today, you will reap the amazing rewards later on. I could literally write hundreds of reasons and benefits of why you must build a physique you'll enjoy and be proud of for years to come. I've personally experienced and seen with my own eyeballs the doors that can open because I'd acquired a strong, powerful physique. I want this unfair advantage for you! The importance of this is so powerful and life changing it is truly hard to put into words. If you are willing to work hard, you deserve to get the best results possible. You have in your hands the best book ever written on how to grow muscle. I left no stone unturned and everything you need is laid out in an easy to under-stand fashion. All that is required is to be able to read at a 3rd grade level and this book will work wonders for you. Anyone who follows this program and works hard will grow muscle at will. Gone is the frustrating guesswork. Read and re-read each chapter thoroughly to fully grasp the true power of the *Bradbury Muscle Course*. Keep this book on your desk or coffee table and read a few pages a day to keep motivation sky high. Remember, out of sight, out of mind. I know one thing, I just wish I would have had something of this magnitude when I first started lifting weights many years ago. I know, without a shadow of a doubt, you'll experience all these great things by simply reading and applying what you learn from this book. This book is about teaching you how to get and keep getting the results you deserve. This book is also about empowering you with the truth. The honest truth that certain dishonest people, behind closed doors, fear that you will one day find. No more wild goose chases! You will not only receive life-altering results, you will receive them much faster than imaginable! Now let's get to work.

I'm not just a guy selling you a training book. This book is a means to get you the results you desire and I com-pletely stand by my solution. Please feel free to email me anytime at beaubradbury@gmail.com. I would love to hear about your experiences and success with the *Bradbury Muscle Course*. I will personally respond to all emails as soon as possible. Send before and after pictures if you'd like. It is absolutely incredible and motivating to hear about the success people are having. If you don't mind, I would be honored if you would write a quick review on Amazon for this book. Also, you can stay in touch and learn more at the *Bradbury Muscle Course* Facebook page: www.facebook.com/bradburymusclecourse

Make Muscles Great Again!

Sadly, thanks to technology, social pressures, and misleading cultural images muscles have gone the way of the VHS tapes. Almost extinct! Many kids today have a proficiency second-to-none on video game controllers, computers, and handheld devices. Instead of being outside chucking bales of hay, playing sports with friends, being active and building their muscles. Today, our youth spends countless hours being programmed by TV, video games and computers. Nowadays, their image of a man is quickly becoming the "dad bod." This is social weakening and it's time to wake up before it is too late! The natural law is that the STRONGEST SHALL SURVIVE. Imagine, if all electrical power was lost and the food supply was delayed just 45 days. These out-of-shape "dad bods" would be slaughtered when exposed to the rigors of nature. Nature has an unforgiving way of quickly eliminating the weak. It would be comical to see those "dad bods," who get winded walking up a flight of stairs, try to defend and feed their family. It is time to wake up people! Physical fitness is your responsibility to yourself and your loved ones. It is time to make muscles great again and especially your muscles. If you've got kids, or plan on having kids in the future, you must lead from the front. Show them what the real image of man is. A man possesses broad, powerful shoulders. A man has thick, muscular arms connected to bulging forearms. A man develops a wide, strong back and chest from lifting and pressing heavy objects. A man will always have calloused hands and a firm handshake. His legs should be powerfully built to make up the timeless "X" shape of a herculean physique. A man always displays prowess and has a take no prisoners attitude. That is what the real symbol of a man is! A man's image is certainly not a hunched over "dad bod" eating a TV dinner and play- ing video games. This is a call to action for you to be the right symbol for the next generation. They will undoubtably follow and emulate what they see. This is how human nature works. We see, we understand importance

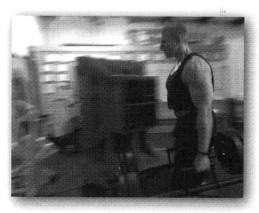

and we attempt to emulate. This mission is bigger than you building a show-stopping physique that will be the envy of your friends, don't worry you'll get that anyways. This is about putting the "MAN" back in MANHOOD! In these overly offensive times, if I've offended you in some way I am not sad and will not feel sorry for you for hurting your feelings. Use your emotional energy to get motivated and put into play the program at the end and find your solu- tion. We all must make it our duty and commit today to make muscles great again!

The *Bradbury Muscle Course* Is Born

The *Bradbury Muscle Course* was designed from the trenches. Working with people just like you day in and day out. We've seen a major shift in the industry towards functional fitness, which I think is great. Functional fitness is a great solution for many people and fits their needs and goals. People who just want to shed some body fat, get a little stronger and healthier for the tasks of everyday life. It has also served as an introduction to fitness for countless people. Some functional fitness programs involve heavy use of a barbell, which is awesome. A pile of free weights and a barbell is superior than an auditorium full of machines any day of the week. Free weights are king! Free weights will always serve as the core of any world-class training program. This book's mission is to teach you how to grow as much muscle as humanly possible. I believe with the sole involvement of compound movements advocated in many functional fitness circles you are leaving loads of potential muscle growth on the table. Compound, multi-joint movements are essential, but I believe and have witnessed they are just a piece of a comprehensive muscle growth program. Take a look at the greats, the giants of the physique world, and it is not by mistake that they also include isolation movements in their training. In addition, it is vital that one must also include isolation movements to refine their physique to build all of their muscles from every possible angle. Once you grasp the importance of including isolation movements, it is also imperative to not forget to always include the basics. Most people totally miss the mark because they do not consistently perform the basic movements (Squat, Bench, Deadlift, Military Press).

In the pages that follow, we will bridge the gap between functional fitness and an extreme muscle building program. My mission is to show you the light to your show-stopping physique you want and deserve. The *Bradbury Muscle Course* is for you, someone who has passion for raw performance, deeply desires muscle mass and razor-sharp definition that will be the talk of town. Once you begin working through this program it will be commonplace for people to ask if you are using steroids. People will begin to bug you for training advice. You will have to buy larger clothing, but your waist will stay the same and in most cases get smaller. Ugly body fat will begin to disappear like magic. Maybe you have been dedicated month in and month out with a certain program, but just haven't acquired the result you've always wanted - a superb, muscular physique. Perhaps, you are just stuck in a rut and are looking for a solution to get back on your A-game. Of course, you might be just starting out and want to be on a bullet train to acquiring an admirable physique. To be clear, this program is a very potent blend of proven strength/power strategies coupled with the main focus of growing muscle tissue (hypertrophy). If your goal is to earn large boulders for shoulders, a massive and wide chest, powerful arms and big wheels that can run through a brick wall, trust me you're in the right place. Not to mention, a thick, strong back that will deadlift piles of iron with ease. If you desire all of this without illegal steroids this book is right up your alley.

Being involved in this field for several years now, I've watched the industry rapidly change so much. You really can't blame a guy for constantly searching for the next magic bullet. I, admittedly, have blindly followed trends and philosophies in hopes of finding superior size and strength. A vision I have had for myself ever since the first time I looked through one of my Dad's muscle magazines he had laying around the house when I was young. That magazine, undoubtably, changed my life. It got me into action and lead to many incredible opportunities that wouldn't have occurred otherwise. I like the common muscle magazines for that reason and am forever grateful. However, I began to notice that the more magazines I read things became more and more confusing. Literally, hundreds of different techniques and six week plans that left me feeling disarrayed. I felt like I had no idea where all this lifting was heading. This ultimately lead to me becoming a freelance exercise programmer at age 17 in a single car garage with my buddy Jared.

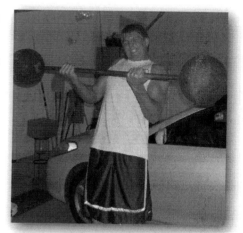

*18 years old on spring
break in La Jolla, CA
Curling a beautiful relic of a barbell*

The logic was let's do Ronnie's massive back routine and Arnold's legendary arm protocol. Scary I know, but by golly it actually worked! Reflecting back, it was pretty amazing. We both transformed our bodies in life changing ways in just six months before we headed off to Lubbock, TX for college. This training period set the stage for a better future. The trouble is, that the crazy mashing of the flavor of the week program in the muscle magazine worked okay for a couple beginner 17-18 year olds, however, it was never optimal and didn't work for long. Let's get one thing clear, when you are a rank beginner to exercise literally anything will work for awhile. You can ride a bicycle and your squat will go up. Add into this we were 17-18 years old, the most anabolic time of our life. My money is on that we were the perfect age, training level and kind of lucked out with our slot machine programming. I have since learned it is just not that simple for more advanced trainees and people who are little older. Again, at that time and circumstances our shotgun approach did work and we were in a single car garage with a very basic weight set and plenty of heat from the hot Texas sun.

After all that, I went off to college at Texas Tech. During my time there I was so very fortunate to have the chance to try out and earned a walk on opportunity for the sport of football. I was so happy to receive this incredible learning experience of participating and enduring a truly comprehensive strength and conditioning program.

Our program was carefully designed by one of the best strength and conditioning coaches in the nation alongside his world-class staff. This whole new experience was a huge eye opener for me. I soon realized that there is much more to this stuff than simply running to the mailbox to get your magazine and making a copy of your favorite bodybuilder's new routine. Each athlete had their own prescribed weights and reps that we were supposed to successfully complete. There was a definite sense of purpose to what we were doing. Some days were easier than others and it all worked together very well. Sadly, I must admit, it worked much better than the magazine Russian roulette. This experience was all it took for me to decide this would become my life's work. I changed my major to Exercise Sciences and began my quest to master the art of this very complex subject. However, I do not truly believe you can fully master anything. I believe learning should never stop and that is especially true in this field. You simply cannot afford to ever stop learning. Your philosophy should evolve into better and better programs over time. I believe you must closely analyze a new idea with an open mind, give it a fair shake and then decide if it works or not. Then you simply take the good from the experience and discard the bad. At Texas Tech University, Exercise Sciences fell under the umbrella of the College of Arts and Sciences. This is for good reason. I believe a superior training program is as much scientific as it is an art. One without the other and the program will be average at best.

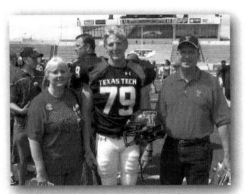

Photo with my parents after the 2008 red & black spring game

Towards the tail-end of my college career, I learned of an emerging fitness trend that has, at the time of the writing of this book, become very mainstream. Constantly searching for the holy grail of training, I jumped in with both feet. The extreme conditioning and heavy influence of going hard and fast every workout was quite addicting I must say. This fast and furious functional fitness program stoked my competitive fire at first. I trained with this method solely with my wife for several years. We also have trained and continue to train many clients to great overall results at our gym using these very methods. I do truly believe if you are looking for a good general physical preparedness and an improved conditioning level this style of program can be a great solution. Without exception, this high speed functional fitness must always be executed in a safe manner or you will get hurt. It always provides tons of variety, so you won't get bored and will stay entertained. It also will cause you to lose lots of scale weight. Personally, I went from around 250lbs and dropped down to just below 190lbs. This style of exercise contains dozens of different movements and most workouts contain a "for time" component, which can be very motivating. I have used these methods with many of my clients throughout the years and it has helped them achieve an awesome general physical preparedness, which is exactly what it is intended to accomplish. Using this particular style of functional fitness you will learn compound movements and will build your conditioning that will prepare you for anything you may encounter in life. This book focuses on achieving extreme lean muscle growth and is in no way an attempt to discredit functional fitness. I have seen this type of functional fitness change many lives for the better with my own eyeballs. Also, performed correctly and supervised by a qualified, experienced fitness professional at all times this program can be a safe endeavor. The reason I bring this all up is because it plays a major role in my journey to create the *Bradbury Muscle Course*. To provide clarity to the reader that if you want an extremely muscular body that is shredded to bits follow this book's program. On the contrary, if you want an all-around fitness that will improve your health functional fitness may be your gig. I am not bashing one for the other. Truly, there is a time and a place for any style of exercise and/or training.

The long pilgrimage back to my roots began one day when I woke up and decided that I missed doing bench press. Honestly, I missed it bad as it was always a staple movement in my pre-functional fitness years. So, on a whim, I decided to see how much I could bench press for a one rep max. This is a very natural thing to do when you are curious about how strong you really are. I started to warm up and quickly became utterly shocked and bewildered! While working up I reached 225lbs, which is a weight I was able to bench 21 times in a row in college. On that day it felt like I was trying to pry a forklift off my chest! At the end of the dismal experiment, it was concluded that I could not even come close to bench press 300lbs for the first time since being 18 years old! This experience had opened my eyes. I became quite disgusted. My bodyweight had plummeted to a thin and lanky sub 190lbs. Which is pretty light considering I am between 6'3" and 6'5" depending on which convenient store I am walking out of. My only guess was that I was so caught up in performing certain workouts with a faster (PR) time, I had completely lost touch with exactly how much strength and muscle was sloughing away. Pictures don't lie and I looked at a photograph (actual photo below) after completing a 5K and looked like I did as a freshman in high school. Skinny and weak compared to what I used to look like. Depression and frustration sadly became a reality. I truly felt like I had lost my identity. During this time, I would almost have to convince people that I even lifted weights and worked out. Whereas in college people would come up to me literally bugging me for lifting advice, programs and even asking if I used steroids (which I've never used illegal steroids). Back then I was one of the big men on campus. Now I seemed to have regressed all the way back to where I was when I started the day I first looked at my dad's muscle magazine. Reality hit me hard square in the face. I was lost. I desperately had to make a change.

My response was that I became a learning machine. I became extremely motivated to figure out how to grow muscle as fast as humanly possible without drugs. My wife and I over the years have spent in excess of $10,000 just on seminars pertaining to training, diet and exercise. Thousands more on continuing education for our professional certifications we hold. Personally, I have spent thousands on training books and programs. Old school, new school, it doesn't matter I've read it then applied the material. I trashed the bad ideas that didn't work and only kept the ideas that worked the best. My mission was to create

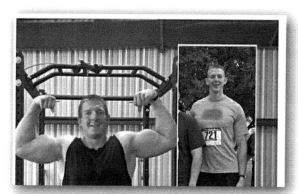

Personally, using the Bradbury Muscle Course strategies, I packed on over 40 pounds of lean muscle completely drug free. I got back to my muscle building roots and it feels great!

the most comprehensive muscle growing program ever. I believe it has been done and it is presented in the following pages in an easy to grasp format. Personally, I have packed on over 40lbs of lean muscle, drug-free, using these exact strategies. My clients that have chosen the route to focus solely on muscle and strength gains have also seen exceptional results. Most of what I am presenting is also backed by the scientific community, however, I will not bore you with listing many different studies on each technique or strategy. Also, please understand many "studies" are skewed to the benefit of the company looking to sell a product or the guy pushing his "new training secret." Most studies are performed on untrained, college kids who just happened to sign up to participate.

Remember, when someone is untrained or is a rank beginner literally anything will work to increase strength and muscle at first. Doing a bear crawl protocol could lead to a bench press increase of a significant percentage. However, you and I both know that doing a bunch of bear crawls is not the optimal way to boost your bench. You must be very vigilant and cautious if you are into believing studies. It is my guarantee to you that I will also strive to continue to learn and apply to improve on the *Bradbury Muscle Course* in the future. As of right now, this is the very best I've got and it will, undoubtably, give you jaw-dropping results if you will simply work hard and follow the program.

Understanding the *Bradbury Muscle Course*

I've always been a big believer in the bottom-line. Is what I am doing providing dynamic results or not? Plain and simple, if it doesn't deliver results it shouldn't exist. Nobody has time to settle for anything less than the best. Although many, if not all, of the ideas presented here are strongly supported by scientific studies somewhere in the world of academia that is not the point or focus of this book. I will not bore you with study after study supporting my claims. If you want to geek out and want studies you can dig them up. This book is solely about growing muscle and teaching you exactly how to do it quickly. This is a "how to" instructional book. The information is to be presented in a format that anyone with a third grade reading level can fully comprehend and apply immediately with ease. As it's commonly said, the proof is in the pudding. I have zero doubt these methods will work wonders for you as they have for countless others. There is science backing these methods, however, this is not a science book. This book shows you how to grow muscle at will step by step. There are numerous people just like you that have maximized their physique using these methods. I, myself, have seen it with my own eyes and witnessed it happen to my own body and the bodies of others. This stuff flat-out works and there is zero unnecessary fluff to fill in lines. The *Bradbury Muscle Course* will work for any human being on the planet. All you have to do is put in the effort required and follow the program to a "T." Imagine, what if I told you that a program truly existed that would maximize your musculature and the musculature of anyone on earth. Wouldn't you want to know about it? Wouldn't you like to find your way out of the discombobulating darkness and into the truth and the light? Imagine, no more worry and anguish of not knowing for sure if what you are doing is even going to work or is it just a waste of precious time and energy. Imagine, attacking the weights everyday with 100% confidence that you are on the fast track to results. Meanwhile, everyone else is slugging along in a beat up Gremlin hatchback in bumper-to-bumper traffic. You will be flying high above speeding to your destination aboard a private jet. If you don't know what a Gremlin is, it just means you are young and a quick internet search will suffice.

The *Bradbury Muscle Course* is delivered to you in a one-of-a-kind "plug and play" format. While most books, publications and articles on training just give you "sample" workouts or routines that may or may not have worked for some guy somewhere, our program is quite the opposite. The *Bradbury Muscle Course* is precise and delivered in such a way that there is zero confusion. There are other run of the mill programs that often leave you confused and wondering if it is the right program for you. I've been there and this situation can be extremely frustrating! You may be attempting to work through a "sample" workout program that was designed for <insert any name here>. Unknown to you, that guy may very well spend thousands per month on pharmaceuticals to enhance his performance and recovery. You may be just a college kid who just worked a couple extra night shifts to save up and buy a jug of protein and creatine. It doesn't take a rocket scientist to figure out this is a bad idea and for certain is not an optimal approach. Now, I do believe that we are all different. Some people are taller than others. Some people have more favorable genetic factors than others when it comes to training. Snarky naysayers will say that a "one size fits all" or "cookie cutter program" won't work. My rebuttal to that claim is wouldn't you agree all humans are pretty much made up from the same stuff (cells, tissues, water etc)? If you cut your finger it bleeds red blood. If you take a 90mph fastball to the back, it will hurt and then a bruise will develop. If you touch a hot stove you will feel pain and your finger will form a burn. On the flip side, wouldn't you agree that if you properly stimulate your muscle tissues and cells, they will respond and grow? If you train certain movements and add weight in a sensible, progressive fashion you will get stronger. If you fuel your body with sound nutrition, you will look and perform better. Keep in mind that this program is about growing your muscles. Muscle tissue adapts to proper training by getting bigger and stronger. This program will work for you and anyone who diligently executes the program in a disciplined manner. From the young gun looking to turn heads on spring break. To the 80 year-old looking to maximize their muscle mass to maintain independent living. This will work wonders for both instances and everyone in between. It is undeniable that what works, WORKS!

The S.A.I.D. Principle

The *Bradbury Muscle Course* roots from what is called the S.A.I.D. Principle. This acronym stands for Specific Adaption to Imposed Demands. In layman's terms, this means that the body will adapt in exact accordance to the demands you place upon it. The human body is an amazingly adaptive creature and can respond to almost any adversity. People have said that if they lose their eyesight due to blindness that their other senses perform at a much higher level to compensate. That in itself shows how truly adaptable our bodies are. The S.A.I.D. Principle is the king kong of all training principles and sadly many people miss the boat by not adhering to it closely. Wouldn't you agree if you wanted to become a professional football player that you must practice countless hours on the game of tennis? Hell no! If you agreed that this was optimal they may take you to a safe place to cool off. While tennis and football do share a few similarities, like agility and hand-eye coordination, they are also completely different games. Can you imagine a tennis player trying to shoot the A-gap in a pro football game? On the flip-side, can you imagine a burly 320lb offensive lineman attempt to hit a delicate drop shot that tags the line? It is a no-brainer that there exists big differences in these two sports. Now that we can all agree on the idiocy that playing baseball everyday will not lead you to win the Tour De France next year we can move on to how all this affects training and program design. As crazy as it sounds, many people unknowingly attempt this play baseball to become an elite cyclist mindset with their training! This is simply from mass confusion and misleading sales tactics. The truth is if you follow the S.A.I.D. Principle and apply it's power to your endeavor you will drastically improve on exactly what you are wanting to improve on. Please understand there is always a few trade offs. If you sacrifice and solely focus on becoming exceptional at a specific endeavor other areas may suffer. If you want to get super strong, you may not want to go strike out on a marathon anytime soon. If you want to build maximal muscle any kind of long, slow endurance activities will be absolutely detrimental to your progress. As amazing as your body is, it only has so much recovery ability. You cannot burn the candle at both ends for long. If you do you will surely notice intensity plummet and eventually get injured. The S.A.I.D. Principle is our guiding light amongst all the darkness and confusion out there. <u>Specific</u> <u>Adaption</u> to <u>Imposed</u> <u>Demands</u> let that sink in. This book is titled *Bradbury Muscle Course - A no-nonsense approach for achieving a lean and muscular physique* and it's proven blueprint roots directly from the S.A.I.D. Principle. You bought this book because you want to grow lots of lean muscle. This is not a book on ultra marathons or how to win a 5K. This book's sole focus is muscle tissue growth aka hypertrophy. Our spotlight is on muscle growth and the philosophy it follows will also lead to extremely potent strength gains as well. To receive muscle hypertrophy you must train for it specifically.

The very art of growing muscle is it's own science. Many lost souls are hoping their current program will give them a muscular appearance, but it never will because the program is not giving the body the proper signals. This is identical to the old DOS computers where you had to input commands. If you were off by one letter or a single punctuation mark the computer would do nothing at all. The computer would just sense a user error. The body is the same way. If you don't input the proper command through your training, you will not get the muscle growth you want. You may indeed work extremely hard, sweat a lot and breathe heavy, but you'll never grow any muscle if the code is wrong. This program assures you this will not be the case. This is because of our unwavering adherence to the S.A.I.D. Principle and our laser focus on growing lean muscle tissue and nothing else. I can say with complete confidence that after the 12-week program enclosed you will see and feel a major difference. Imagine, after just 6 months to a year of performing these 12-week cycles how show-stopping your physique will become. You will never have to do another program again. Let's dive into the details of growing muscle!

What is Hypertrophy?

No! Hypertrophy is not a trophy you get for being the most hyper. Good guess though. Since the mission of this book is focused on how to maximize muscle hypertrophy. It is of most importance to clearly define what hypertrophy is. Not only defining it, but also give you the proven philosophy that will give you more of it. Muscle Hypertrophy is defined as the growth and enlargement of muscle cells. Bigger muscle cells equals BIGGER MUSCLES! While evidence is split and inconclusive on the idea of the possibility of increasing the actual number of muscle cells through a theoretical process called hyperplasia. The facts are conclusive that muscle hypertrophy (increase in cell size, not number) does exist. Evidence proves that muscles can grow much larger by maximizing hypertrophy in your training. Hypertrophy, like economics, is one of the rare instances where more is actually better! Once you become interested in building muscle, you really can't build too much. "OMG, I'm all upset because my biceps have grown too big!!" -said no man ever. Unlike most things in life, having too much muscle has zero negative side effects and many positives. There exist many different "theories," methods, and supplements promising the holy grail of supernatural muscle growth. Whenever you have many different possible directions it generates nothing but confusion. My mission is getting you the muscle you desire through a simple, proven approach. No smoke and mirrors here. If you do this program, it will work. It is that simple. There is no reason why you couldn't read, comprehend and apply this information in a matter of a few hours. Then immediately put into action this one-of-a-kind "plug and play" program leading you to muscular dominance. The *Bradbury Muscle Course* lives and breathes by a philosophy that the best physiques in history have always fully understood and applied. If there is really a secret, this is it. Get your pencils ready and write this bad boy down! This basic philosophy is the secret that divides the people who get outstanding results and the poor souls who work hard, but get only marginal results or worse none whatsoever. So what's the big secret? How do I know I won't become one of those poor souls? First off, congratulations since you've got this book in your hands and are reading it you are now amongst the enlightened few. You are going to build slabs of lean muscle. Since you might still be asking here is the big secret! This philosophy is not only proven, but it serves as a core principle of this program. It is the undeniable truth that: BIGGER IS STRONGER, STRONGER IS BIGGER!

7

The Big Miss

The contents of this chapter have always weighed heavily on my heart. To fully understand the power of the following words, you must understand how this book was written. This book was fully scribed via a #2 pencil and a notebook. Over the span of many months, going over every detail of this program pulling from years of personal experience and years of experience working with many different clients. I wrote down and documented what worked and what didn't. I was on a mission of one day presenting you a program that delivers unbelievable results that was simple to apply. I was smack dab in the middle of writing the chapter over nutrition when these thoughts began to well up in me, similar to how steam builds in a pressure cooker. I began to recall all of the conversations of the past and remembering all the people I'd seen throughout the years. Many who came to me at a crossroads in their life in regards to health. Many who were beyond frustrated with their current physical condition desperately seeking help. Many others I have never met, but I could witness how their poor fitness was wrecking havoc on their daily lives. The real-life struggle of millions of Americans. They are searching for help and not finding any. Feverishly, I began writing what was coming out of my mind onto the paper immediately instead of fighting the urge to just finish the nutrition chapter and moving on. These feelings and thoughts are divinely meant to be in this book I believe. The words below are written word for word without any editing (uncut version) in that notebook that afternoon:

"This chapter is written way out of place. I am in the middle of writing the nutrition chapter. This is because these thoughts are coming across my heart as I am writing and I feel it is of extreme importance. Please understand how this book was written. I wrote this with a pencil and a notebook. What drove me to do so is unknown, but mainly out of a lack of a book like this available. After buying and reading countless books and articles, I couldn't ever find what I was really looking for. After interacting with many people it become apparent of the mass confusion when it comes to proper training lurking around the fitness industry. It sickens me how people looking for help, will spend big dollars and always go home empty handed. Much of the industry is designed to only make money and, more often than not, fail miserably at delivering actual results. The many different deceitful sales tactics and 2 year contracts that plague the industry has always made me sick to my stomach. Literally ill. Seeing willing, hopeful people go try to get results and be set up to fail from the get-go. The system is failing the mass majority. Our obesity and health crisis continues to climb when at the exact same time the number of gym memberships in America are at the highest ever! This is the big miss. This means the number of gym memberships and the percentage of obesity have both climbed together and both are at the highest level ever right now. Somebody is getting ripped off! It is not working.

With the rise of many "certificate mills" more and more people have entered the industry as a part-time gig. They treat it as a silly hobby and do not grasp the grave importance of their temporary position. After just spending a few dollars and a few hours reviewing a little information and subsequently passing an elementary-level test they now boast to call themselves "trainers" or worse "coaches." Instantly, they foolishly act like they are now highly regarded experts. They are a disgrace to the real professionals who spend literally countless hours studying and becoming a master of their craft, honing their skills every single day. These weekend warriors are, unknowingly, driving groves of participants away from the fitness industry all together. People desperately searching for help, may do their due diligence and interact with a real professional and get mind-blowing results or they may not. The unfortunate souls may deal with an enthusiastic part-timer who hasn't and won't do their due diligence and understand the severity of their position as a "trainer" or "coach." This inevitable end result is a potential future success story that goes home empty handed once again. These part-timers simply do not know what they do not know. Sadly, just another victim who suffered through an unprofessional and frustrating experience that, undoubtably, will leave a foul taste in their mouth regarding the fitness industry. It can and often does get worse. Desperate to find individuality, the under-educated "coach" or "trainer" forces a certain insane workout "challenge", advanced movement, etc on their willing client in hopes of posting the coolest social media video of the day. This kind of idiocy will lead to a severe injury, life-threatening medical problems or worse. It is akin to playing with fire or a dog chasing cars. You know the ending. As disgusting as this is, this is becoming the norm now. This is a tragedy for you, myself, and anyone participating in the industry. This is dangerous, irresponsible and downright sickening. For gyms to make even more money on these poor, misguided souls they get their freshly minted "trainer" in front of a high-paying client immediately. Unbeknownst to the client paying big bucks their new unexperienced "coach" or "trainer" has no clue what they are doing and they're just winging it. To make things worse, in a futile attempt to look smart, they will blindly repeat what they were taught at their short-lived certificate program. Many times they don't even know if it has been proven to be wise advice or not. They just regurgitate what they can scramble to remember, just like a bird vomiting up food to their baby chicks! Don't fall victim to these hucksters.

Believe it or not, it has become common for gyms to barely or not even pay these weekend warrior "trainers" or "coaches." Some just do enough to mess things up for the client, but don't care as long as they are insured their free "coach's" membership. All of this is so the immoral gym can pry more money from your pocket and into theirs. It makes zero sense to pay a high-end price for a low-end product. Now that you've read these words, you my friend are one of the few that have been enlightened! You now have seen the other side of the desk. I believe, more than ever, in the true value of working with an experienced and qualified fitness professional. Trust me, there are many wonderful fitness professionals out there that can help you. However, you must be vigilant and smart! Protect yourself and always do your due diligence when searching for a fitness professional. Do not succumb to sneaky sales tactics and cheaper prices. Always remember you get exactly what you pay for. If something is cheaper it will be a cheaper experience. Diligent research can go along ways in identifying a real professional. Ask to see a portfolio. Ask around for referrals from long-term clients. In all honesty, it is easy to tell a pro from a joe. Make sure they look the part. There are many "trainers" or "coaches" who don't even look like they workout. What a joke! If they can't seem to manage to get results on their own body, what makes you think they will do so for you? Mark my words! This book will not go without its fair share of scrutiny and controversy. These things come with the territory whenever the truth is finally revealed to the masses. People who don't want you to know these truths will throw up their skinny arms in disgust. They will come up with crafty lies and make up stories to ensure their prosperous money scheme isn't exposed. Truly, I fear for you, our nation, and the fitness industry. If things keep going like they are going the masses will just become weaker and weaker. Epidemic levels of sickness, obesity and premature death will continue to rise at alarming rates. Our nation, which used to pride itself on being powerful and hard working, will become crippled and lazy. This book is about making muscles great again, but it's also about re-routing the course. A strong human race make better workers, better protectors and are much less demand on our country. Strong people makes a strong community. Strong communities will make a strong state. Finally, strong states will make a healthy and strong country once again! We must take action now, because sadly the exact opposite is also true. Simply, replace the word "strong" in the preceding sentences to "sick." Make sure you do your part and change your body to be a part of changing your country. The trouble has always been how exactly do we do it? Rampant mass confusion has lead to many people being grossly misguided. So many deceptive and troublesome "ideas" always promising instant results and then simply don't deliver the goods. Many are impossible to sustain and make part of your lifestyle. Many just flat-out do not work! This book's only mission is your results. My philosophy from day one has been about getting people results they desire. Is it safe? Is it smart? Does it work every single time? Does it get people results? These are the questions that must answer "YES" every single time. The ideas presented in the Bradbury Muscle Course have been proven time after time on countless bodies and even my own. Finally, you have in your hands a results-based program provided in an easy to use format. Anyone could literally skip all the reading and go straight to the program in the back and start changing their body for the better immediately. The Bradbury Muscle Course will work for anyone who performs the program with great effort and diligence. This is your solution!"

This is a tough subject to go over with you. However, I want you in the know. I'm tired of hearing stories from innocent people who are getting ripped off and discouraged. Now you are forewarned and know exactly how to maneuver and avoid a costly mistake. At this point, I encourage you to go back and re-read the "Make Muscles Great Again!" chapter. If those words don't get you jacked up to pump iron, you better rush to the hospital and get your pulse checked.

The Solution: Build More Muscle

Groves of people every year decide they want to get into shape. They want to "lose weight" and "tone up." The sad part is the majority fail and fail miserably in their endeavor. 99% of the time is due to a lack of understanding what exactly they are trying to accomplish. So many times in an effort to improve their physique they will start crash diets and endurance-type training. They start running or using cardio machines. In all likelihood, this is probably what their parents did when they tried to lose weight and probably failed also. The trouble is they don't fully grasp what they are trying to accomplish. When you go about a successful physical transformation you must put all of your focus on muscle first. It must be your top priority! Adding lean muscle mass boosts your metabolism. Lean muscle mass burns up calories throughout the day. Muscle burns more calories at rest and during exercise. It is common sense that if you add lean muscle your physique will look different. Working to rid the body of extra fat and adding lean muscle causes your muscle to show. The fat melting away will show off your muscles by giving them definition. Most people would agree that a muscular physique with very low body fat is more aesthetically pleasing to the eye. Even ladies who are looking to get into shape want to have muscle tone and that takes a dedicated approach to building muscle. High intensity cardio can be beneficial for getting leaner, however it must not take the priority over focused muscle building. Long, slow cardio activities will simply strip off any extra lean muscle leaving you in an even worse predicament. Be vary cautious when using BMI or height/weight charts to determine your health. Muscle is much denser and weighs more than fat, therefore you could have less than 10% body fat and carry and lot of lean muscle and be considered obese on these charts. On the flip side, you could have a "skinny fat" person who has minimal muscle and a high body fat percentage, however, their total body weight puts them in the "healthy" range. Even though it doesn't take a rocket scientist to figure out that a weak person with a higher body fat percentage isn't really the picture of health. The best way to know if you are moving in the right direction is by measuring your percentage of body fat periodically and tracking progress. Our mission is the long term winning solution of building as much lean muscle as possible and reducing body fat over time. We do this by focusing on muscle growth in training and by reducing our caloric intake a sensible amount. As your body changes you will see results in the mirror and on your body fat percentage. There are many ways to measure your body fat percentage. Some methods are more accurate than others. You can use skin calipers, underwater weighing, bod pod, bioelectrical impedance devices and so on. There are many choices. Anyone can learn how to use a skin caliper and they are fairly accurate depending on the user. Personally, I use the AccuMeasure® Fitness 3000 Body Fat Caliper. It is easy to learn and you simply measure one area. The best part is that you can do it quickly and accurately (with practice) by yourself in the privacy of your own home. Another great method is looking into the mirror. You can see when your body fat is getting lower and muscles are building. Some people need to see numbers and they will want to use a caliper or some other body fat percentage measuring method. If you want a permanent transformation, you need to focus on increasing muscle and shedding excess fat. If you are wanting to lose weight, do not get upset if at first you weigh and see that you've gained scale weight. The scale can be your enemy by creating doubt. Remember muscle is much more dense and weighs more than fat. You could pack on 5 pounds of solid lean muscle, lose 4 pounds of pure fat and show on the scale that you gained a net of 1 pound. Imagine how different your body would look if you gained 15 pounds of lean muscle and lost 15 pounds of pure ugly fat. However, the scale would tell you that you weigh the same as when you started! Even though you now look completely different. Too many people are mislead because of the bathroom scale. If you are a numbers person find a method to measure body fat percentage and stick to that. Our program is designed to build incredible amounts of lean muscle. Getting your diet and calories dialed in will control body fat levels. I believe you should work to achieve a physique that is strong, muscular and have a visible six pack all year. Our program will help you accomplish this as fast as possible. By following the diet guidelines and working hard on the *Bradbury Muscle Course* you cannot fail. You will build muscle. Your body fat will disappear. You will be stronger than ever. Just understand the golden ticket is building muscle through sound resistance training. Do not end up like the masses and get on a health kick just to end up even fatter in the long haul. Start building today. Most people fail because they do not know and understand what you just learned. Masses of people get on a treadmill and the latest fad diet. They strip all their muscle off and unknowingly put their body into starvation mode. They increase their body's ability to store body fat. Muscle is no longer there to help speed up their metabolism. Their diet is too severe to become a habit and eventually they quit. The weight they lost comes back and most times they become fatter than ever before. This is due to improper diet and removing lean muscle tissue. The end result is the highest body fat percentage ever, slowest metabolism ever, and worst of all the least amount of lean muscle mass ever! It is simply a losing approach. These goofy tactics are the reason why you know people who are always on a diet, but their weight is on a roller coaster. They are the definition of a "yo yo" dieter. This leaves you very unhealthy and weak. Do not ever take this route. Commanding physiques are built with resistance training that increases lean muscle. This boosts your metabolism to start stripping fat. Over time your lean mass increases exponentially and your body fat percentage drops lower and lower. Your friends can't even recognize you. People can't believe how you are so muscular and defined. They start wondering if you are using steroids or something. Just get it in your head that it all starts with muscle. Focus solely on building muscle and your body starts changing right away. Don't believe me? Go on ahead and hit the treadmill and eat grapefruits and rice cakes and see what happens. Increasing lean muscle mass is the secret of the best physiques on the planet. This is true for both men and women. Work hard to grow and maintain lean muscle and losing fat will become easier and easier with time. If you are serious about changing your look drastically, do not fall victim to distractions and fall off the wagon. Give your training and nutrition 6 months of very strict discipline and you will be appalled what the *Bradbury Muscle Course* will do for you.

Philosophy

I am a huge believer in principles. When you get off track it is easy to refer back to your guiding principles. They will always set you straight. It's been said that circumstances may change, but principles never change. Personally, I got tired of seeing people getting taken advantage of by con artists. Countless people falling into the trap of deceptive marketing that made them believe that what they desired could come easy and fast. Instead of just sitting on the sideline shaking my head in disgust, I decided to do something about it. What you hold in your hands now is my solution. I know if I have someone's undivided attention I can get them an incredible physical transformation. Before this book, those incredible transformations were reserved only for my clients who are teachable, disciplined and apply my methods. I wanted to create a way to reach the masses with the truth. I was so tired of seeing people get jacked around, so I decided to write this book to fix this issue. The issue is that people get hit with so many possible "quick fixes." The problem is they don't work. I want to teach you how to get jaw dropping results as quickly as possible and how to improve on them over time. Don't get me wrong, earning a stellar physique is hard work! You must work extremely hard and give it time. This will not be easy. However, it will be worth it. When I began writing I knew I must have a set of principles to keep me headed into the right direction. These 7 principles apply today and will apply 100 years from now.

THE 7 PRINCIPLES OF THE *BRADBURY MUSCLE COURSE*

1)   There is no such thing as a "quick fix" that actually works

The number one problem people encounter is falling for the marketing trap of fast and easy. I wanted to make it clear that the fast and easy approach does not work. If it does work it will only be a temporary fix and in time you'll regress back to your formal self or worse. Building a strong, muscular physique with minimal body fat is truly a lifestyle. You must understand it will be hard work and it will take time. Anything worth having requires hard work. You must prepare yourself for extreme discipline and hard work. A quote to live by...

"the only place success comes before work is in the dictionary."

-VINCE LOMBARDI

2) Resistance training is the holy grail for a transformation

You decide you are willing to sacrifice and work hard to build a superbly muscular physique. Your program must be a resistance training program. There is no exceptions. Even if you need to lose 100 pounds of fat, your program must be a resistance training program. A comprehensive resistance training program will do wonders for any physique. You will build lean muscle, melt fat and get healthier. Your program must include compound and isolation movements with free weights. Sure machines can be a great supplement, but the majority of your training should be done with free weights. Even many weight loss experts who take morbidly obese people and help them become healthy and fit agree that resistance training is a integral part of healthy weight loss. To become extremely muscular and extremely lean resistance training is your best friend.

3) Results are the name of the game

I'm a bottom line guy and if something is not producing I don't have time for it. This principle is the main reason why I wrote this book and designed the *Bradbury Muscle Course*. Over the span of many years, I developed a program that delivered results and I wanted to get it into your hands. In my quest, I tried many different training programs. Some worked okay and others were a waste of time. I wanted a results-based program that provided visible results for everyone. Everything in this book is in there for one simple reason… it provides you results. More muscle, less fat and insane strength increases is the result you will get if you just work hard and stay disciplined.

4) Strive for safety and longevity

It's never made a bit of sense to me that people get hurt working out. If the goal is to better yourself and build your body up, why on earth are you thrashing yourself with insane challenges and goofy movements? While it is true that anyone can get injured on any exercise, it is also true that you can minimize risk by being smart. With built in recovery periods and sensible progressions it is my belief that people can train at a very high intensity and do so with a remarkably low risk of injury. Our program uses periodization techniques to ramp up intensity in a smart manner. You are responsible to increase load sensibly by making logical jumps in weight (see art of progression chapter). This program is about building up all of your muscles which makes a leaner, healthier body. This is not some goofy "challenge" or "make you puke!" endeavor. This is an extreme muscle building program that specializes in physique transformations. We also train in a safe and smart manner. There is no reason why you can't push yourself and start growing today and for years to come.

5) Always value aesthetics

There are some people who scoff at people who obviously value training for aesthetics. Physical aesthetics should be the bullseye of your training program. A strong body is healthier than a weak one. A lean body is healthier than a fat one. A muscular body is healthier than a frail one. If you add those up, you will come up with an aesthetically pleasing human being. It is impossible to be strong, muscular and lean and not totally own the beach. Most people I have encountered looking to start training want to look and feel better. I gear my programs for dynamic visible results. This may not align with everyone and that is okay. Some people accept looking average. I consider myself a physique transformation specialist. My mission is to help you pack on muscle, strip ugly fat and get stronger. I am not really into being your babysitter or coming up with "entertainment" workouts. I want you to get the results you came for. End of story. Most people desire jaw dropping results and the *Bradbury Muscle Course* delivers the goods.

6) Nutrition trumps training

You can have the best program in the world, but if your diet is lousy you will not get the results you desire. I believe wholeheartedly that the *Bradbury Muscle Course* is the best program in the world for building rock hard muscle, ridding body fat, and drastically improving strength. I would be lying to you if I said you didn't have to worry about eating right. You must be vigilant with your nutrition and supplement use. You can't eat right for a week or two and give up. You must eat right, day in day out, forever if you are serious about achieving an uncommon physique. It must become a lifestyle. It has been said that your body reflects today what your diet contained six months ago. If you are hellbent on extreme results, you simply cannot afford to make mistakes with your diet. Give yourself time and stay strong. Mark my words, nutrition will make or break you! I have noticed with my clients doing the exact same program there are the ones who listen, eat right and use supplements as advised and there are those who simply don't. They both work hard in workouts, but it is incredible the vast difference in their results. Remember, they are doing the same exact training programs! One earns a jaw dropping transformation and the other doesn't because of poor eating habits. One stays strong and disciplined day in and day out. The other binges on beer, pizza and desserts on the weekends. If you make proper eating a lifestyle, muscle will come much faster and fat will disappear easier. One of my favorite quotes to live by comes from the late, great Jack LaLanne…

"Exercise is king. Nutrition is queen. Put them together and you've got a kingdom."

7) The big secret is persistence

It is human nature to quit something that is hard. It is the way we are wired. It is my estimate that over 95% of human physiques are average at best. I'm not a big secret guy, but if there is a secret it is persistence! The majority will quit. The uncommon will persist without exception. Trust me there are going to be days when you will want to quit and throw in the towel. If you are serious about earning results, you are going to have to stick it out. That is the bottom line. Worst case scenario, walk away for one week and think about if you really want to quit. Most times this is all it takes to get fired up and back on track. You should remember why you started this endeavor in the first place. If earning an extremely muscular physique was easy, everyone would have one. If everyone has one it becomes undesirable. The discipline and effort required is what makes it so special. Muscle never lies. The majority start out strong and usually fizzle out within 8 weeks. If you don't want to be average, you must persist and push through. The *Bradbury Muscle Course* is designed to help you persist by utilizing growth weeks to let your body fully recover and let your mind recharge for the next intense 3 weeks. When you are tired it is never wise to make a decision because your emotions will get the best of you. The most productive people on the planet avoid making any big decision after 3PM, because they know that making a decision when tired will be a mistake. I'm not saying that persisting without exception will be an easy task, however our program is specially designed to avoid burnout and accumulated fatigue. It will be much easier for you to use persistence when you feel fresh and full of vigor every training day. Write this timeless quote down!

"Patience, persistence and perspiration make an unbeatable combination for success"

- NAPOLEON HILL

Part 2: Methods of the Madness

Congratulations you are about to enter Part 2: Methods of the Madness. By now you should be chomping at the bit to start changing your body by building muscle. How exactly does one go about building lots of muscle as fast as possible? No worries my friend part 2 will make the complex, simple for you. You will learn why we do what we do and how to do it. This portion of the book is all the nuts and bolts you'll ever need to craft a commanding physique. Building maximum muscle is not an easy endeavor, in fact most people fail miserably as you've seen. You will have all the tools and knowledge you'll ever need. Most importantly, you'll know exactly how to implement them to make your muscles grow like weeds. One theme of this book is showing you the truth presented with short, concise chapters. Personally, I do not like long, drawn out, boring chapters as it seems to cause a lack of focus. If you cannot read a chapter in a few minutes it is too long in my opinion. I like to get to the point fast and get you all the information you need to be successful and move on. I'm not here to entertain you with cool stories. I am here to show you how to make your muscles grow! Let's get down to business.

10

Burly Basics

Any effective muscle building program must involve getting stronger on the basic movements. If the program does not include the basics, go run because you'll be scrawny anyways and at least you might see some wildlife. The basics are what are rightfully referred to as the BIG THREE and include the squat, bench press, and deadlift. Building up to a substantial total in these lifts are what set the men from the boys. Many pencilneck "experts" will ridicule these movements. These claims come from sheer ignorance, a lack of ability to lift respectable numbers in these lifts, and/or a futile attempt to sell some goofy exercise device to hang your clothes on down the road in your closet. Don't believe these goofballs for one second if you want to build muscle. If you are going to a bar fight and you have to pick one friend to bring along, would you take the guy with a 600lb deadlift or the guy with a 185lb deadlift? I know I am taking my new best friend with the 600lb deadlift every single time! The amount you can lift on the big three is the gauge of your overall prowess. The big three is also proficient for packing on slabs of muscle. They are your foundation to build upon. I first heard this quote from Dr. Fred Hatfield aka Dr. Squat at one of his seminars, "you cannot shoot a canon out of a canoe!" This is timeless wisdom as the original quote seems to date back to 1800's naval warfare. The big three will turn you from a flimsy canoe into a massive battleship ready to take on any adversary. Just the simple act of performing these movements stimulates tons of muscle fibers in your body. This naturally increases favorable muscle building hormone levels for even more growth. The big three also improve full body strength drastically, this allows more weight to be used on other movements including all isolation movements. All this means for you is just more and more muscle gain. The big three are truly the forefathers of many other great movements. They have brothers, sisters and even cousins. For example, if you have a massive squat you will be able to use more weight on say Bulgarian split squats to pack on even more quad muscle. The big three is the MVP in our program. These multi-joint, compound movements have proven to work for decades and make up the core of our extreme hypertrophy program.

11

Isolation Works

If a prison is having trouble with a certain inmate they put them into a isolation cell and it solves the problem. I digress, back to talking about how to build yourself BIG muscles. In some circles, isolation movements are like the boogey-man! In recent times, isolation movements have gotten a bad wrap claiming they are not "functional." Personally, I think this is a goofy ideology and is not inline at all with building maximal muscle. If isolation movements are in fact not "functional" I propose a simple "functional" test! The claim is a bicep curl is not a "functional" movement. So would this mean that curling your arm is not "functional," therefore not important to sustain life? This is starting to get a little crazy. Why not duct-tape a 2"x4" board from wrist to armpit and try to survive for 3 days? Let that sink in. The board will not allow your arm to bend a single inch since arm curls aren't "functional." With your arms straight it would be quite the challenge to eat, drink, and wipe your a**. This could get messy! If you want to try this experiment go ahead at your own risk. To save yourself much trouble just get it into your head that isolation movements are not the devil and actually work quite well. They will even help your "functional" movement performances improve drastically! We all know that a chain is only as strong as it's weakest link. This timeless statement can be applied directly to your training. Say you have a weak and lagging body part, only through isolation movements can you isolate that area to bring it up to speed. Picture this, you are trying to get your very first chin-up. The chin-up involves your back and biceps. Let's say your biceps are scrawny and weak. You decide to build them up to 18" by implementing the bicep curl variations in the *Bradbury Muscle Course*. After you accomplish this goal, chin-ups are now a breeze. Cranking out ten to fifteen reps becomes the norm. On the flip-side, you'd have to be looney to think that doing bicep curls wouldn't at least help you to get your first chin-up. You have made your whole chain stronger, by making every single link stronger. Only through isolation movements is this possible. Everyone wants to build a show stopping set of arms. It is true that you can build decent arms without isolations, however we aren't after decent. The truth is to build extraordinary guns you must do direct arm work. While it is also true that deadlifts work your traps to a certain degree, they do not work them to the same magnitude as a gut-wrenching heavy set of shrugs in the hypertrophy range of 8-15 reps. If you don't believe me, try it! See for yourself.

What exactly is an isolation movement or is there such a thing? Generally, an isolation movement is referred to as a single joint movement like a bicep curl or a lateral raise for deltoids (shoulders). Muscles are meticulously assembled in groups. We say quads or quadriceps, but that is actually four large muscles and many others assisting in their function and movements. It is my belief that there is no such thing as a true isolation movement. This is because there are numerous muscles working alongside the targeted muscle or as synergists to perform any movement. For the sake of simplicity and to minimize confusion, we will stick to the name isolation movements even though we know working only one single muscle is taboo. Since, we understand the fact that many muscles are involved in performing even the simplest of moves. The *Bradbury Muscle Course* utilizes isolation movements in precise proportion to compound movements to spark maximum muscle growth and to fortify all links in your chain. The isolation movements build on the foundation of the big three and the other foundational movements. For superb muscle growth, you must have both in precise amounts. They are like peanut butter and jelly. Isolation movements will generally be worked in the 8-15 rep range which is known to spike muscle hypertrophy. We will also focus on many sets of 11 with the isolation movements. More on the magic of 11's later on. All past giants in the strength and physique arena have included isolation movements in their program and you should too! Don't be left behind.

The Ultimate Hybrid

In my treacherous quest for the ultimate muscle growth blend to deliver maximal musculature coupled with a strong side effect of strength gains, I believe I've made it. There is really nothing quite like the perfect blend. Just the right amount of chocolate protein powder, peanut butter, water and the precise amount of ice and a perfect blend is born! It tastes amazing and goes down smooth every time. It must be precise and perfect. Too much or too little of any one ingredient and your blend goes to hell in a handbasket in no time flat. With the *Bradbury Muscle Course*, you have in your hands the pinnacle of master blends. The precise amount of compound movements and isolation movements. Perfectly crafted with precise amounts of volume of reps and sets. Set up in an exact use of periodization that will never leave you feeling burned out or crippled with overtraining. Instead, you will always feel great day in and day out to push the limits of your intensity. All of this is presented in a revolutionary "plug and play" fashion. Every workout is displayed in such a manner you don't have to think. Even in such detail down to the very last rep. In other words, all the work is done for you. All you have to do is attack each workout with great effort and record the results in your workout log. Imagine, how much time you will save by not having to try to figure out what workout to do and how many reps and sets to perform. More importantly, wondering around thinking "is this even going to work?" With this program you've got it made in the shade with lemonade. I've done all of the investigating and trial and error for you to come up with a truly

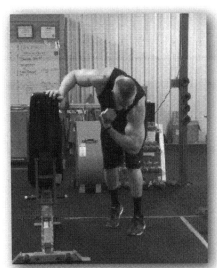

A precise combination of compound and isolation movements will put your muscles into a growth frenzy!

effective and life altering program. I only wish this book was available when I started lifting. It would have been nice to have avoided all of the rookie mistakes and failed training regimens. You are one fortunate soul and the many fine details of the *Bradbury Muscle Course* are explained in the following chapters. Master these and you will master the art of growing muscle.

Muscle Growth Triad

When one is attempting to grow as much muscle as possible there must be a specific aim to do so. Too many times people are unsatisfied with their results because their training program is too predictable or has way too much variance. Your training must focus solely on the task at hand. I believe that extreme muscle growth can and will be achieved at will if you always adhere to the triad: The Muscle Growth Triad. The sum of the three critical parts make up a whole and a chain is only as strong as it's weakest link. This is why our program is superior. Our program uses elements of the Muscle Growth Triad in a balanced approach to deliver maximal results. Our revolutionary Muscle Growth Triad is made of three critical parts: *Strength, Hypertrophy, & Shock*. As mentioned several times in this book, to build maximal muscle a person must also become stronger in the process. The stronger you become on the basic movements, you automatically become stronger on the muscle-specific movements. A guy that can deadlift 500lbs will be able to use more weight on say a T-bar row than a guy with a 215lb deadlift. This is why it is imperative for strength to have a spot on the triad. The second spot on the triad belongs to hypertrophy. Hypertrophy is a scientific word that means an increase in the size of muscle cells. Kind of a big deal if you are looking to build big muscles. It should go without saying, but if you sincerely desire a defined, muscular physique you must train specifically for muscle growth. Hypertrophy specific training protocols must make up a major part of any effective muscle building program. Proper hypertrophy training will utilize a rep range between 8-15 reps and have shorter rest periods. This induces an extreme muscle pump. Where nutrient-rich blood gorges the muscle stretching out the fascia. All these biological phenomenons lead to bigger muscles! Last but certainly not least is shock. The human body is an extremely adaptive organism. Which is great for survival. However, your training program must always outsmart the body. If you do the same thing

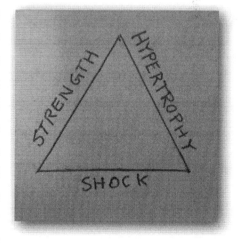

over and over again the body knows what is coming. If your body becomes too familiar with your training, your results will start to fall off into the grand canyon. You must shock your muscles to keep them off balance. By using the intensity techniques outlined in the the *Bradbury Muscle Course* you will do just that. Our program has built in shock methods that will keep your muscles growing and growing. Imagine, if you always do bench presses and then head over to incline presses and then do flys your body will quickly figure out your plan. The body would be shocked if you started with incline presses first and then went to bench presses followed by flys. It would be totally shocked if you did flys first with a cluster protocol, then incline presses and finished it all off with a bench press drop set. Your muscles will literally be shaking and pumped to the max after their shocking experience. This is why shock has the final place on the all important Muscle Growth Triad. Don't be left in the dark with scrawny arms. Put the Muscle Growth Triad into your corner to own the beach.

Rep Ranges for Maximum Muscle

Believe it or not, all types of your muscle fibers can and will grow if stimulated correctly. The fast-twitch fibers grow much larger than the slow-twitch fibers, but nonetheless all fibers can enlarge. To achieve maximal muscle growth you must stimulate as many fibers as possible. Some fibers respond to fast, explosive movement. Others respond to a moderate weight with reps performed more rhythmically. Lastly, some fibers are more endurance oriented and require long, slow sets with very high reps. In this comprehensive muscle building program, most days you will perform 12 or less reps on the core movements and reps between 5-30 on the other movements. However, there will be shock days. So be prepared to see anything. We will leave no stone unturned! When it comes to growing as much muscle as possible you cannot afford to.

How to Perform a Rep

There are two ways to perform a repetition:

1. You can do whatever it takes to move the weight from point A to point B
2. You can focus on feeling the muscle(s) move the weight through the range of motion

There is a time and a place for everything. The two examples above happen in gyms everyday. Example #1 brings to mind maxing out with heavy weights or the sport of powerlifting. Most of the time if the weight is near maximum you cannot even attempt to try to feel your muscles working. Rather, you must strain and give it all you got to get the weight up to finish the rep. Whereas example #2 you think of bodybuilding and physique work. Feeling the muscle working against a moderate load to produce a pump and grow muscles to their maximal size and definition. I am going to stand up on my soap box and say both are correct at the right time. On week 11 of this program you will work up to a 5 rep max (or a 3RM or even a 1RM if you so choose). This is a true test of raw strength and to see how much stronger you are becoming as you go from cycle to cycle. This is vital to do, because it is a precise way to measure your strength gains with little to no error. At that time, you'll instinctively utilize rep example #1 above during maximum efforts and that is wonderful. You are trying to move as much weight as possible from point A to point B to establish a new personal best on your major lifts. Since the aim of this book is to grow as much muscle as possible, rep example #2 must be employed for the bulk of our work. When you focus hard and perform every single rep with a great stretch and a great contraction you will build more muscle. Period. Versus the goofball who's eyes are always bigger than his muscles and grabs too much weight all the time and does a bunch of junky reps. He thinks he impressing his fellow gym goers, instead they are wondering if he suffers from some rare muscle spasm disease and if they should render aid. Don't be that guy. Another glaring problem that exists is the frequent slashing of range of motion (ROM). The weights start to get a little heavy and people are quick to start cutting off range of motion. Unfortunately, taking the path of least resistance is in fact human nature. Never allow yourself to succumb to this level of mediocrity and cut reps off short. You are failing yourself miserably. Not only are you leaving lots of potential muscle on the table, but you are making a complete fool out of yourself. If it is a bench press touch your chest and go up to lockout. On squats go down to parallel or slightly below and stand up all the way. If it is a curl go from straight arms to a full contraction at the top. If you can't do this simple task because the weight is too heavy, then lighten it up a little and do it right. You will never really know if you are getting any stronger unless you always perform full reps religiously.

To be accurately measurable every rep must be exactly the same. If you squat 225 for one full rep and then half squat 700 for one rep, your true 1 rep measurable squat is 225. The moral of the story is commit to doing every rep using the full range of motion.

MAIN POINTS:

1. Focus to achieve a great STRETCH and a great CONTRACTION every single rep.
2. Always perform full RANGE OF MOTION every rep. Never cut reps short.
3. Utilize an all or nothing approach only on maximum efforts focusing on doing whatever it takes to move the bar from point A to point B.

16

Rest Assured

Precise rest in between must be a followed with precision to achieve the proper stimulus and thus results we are looking to achieve. Most people erroneously pay no attention to rest periods and this robs them from their desired results. You must be vigilant and take rest periods seriously and be exact. A simple wristwatch can go along way here. Personally, I use rest breaks to quickly jot down my results from the previous set in my workout log. The allotted rest time allows the body to rejuvenate to blast through the next effort. During the "pump focus" portions you'll notice much shorter rest periods. Shorter rest periods are linked to more muscle growth and an enhanced favorable hormone release. A friendly word of advice, use a pen and paper journal and not your phone. While there are some cool apps to log weights and such, I don't advise it. Your phone can easily turn into a distraction. It can also give people the wrong sense of what you are doing. Phones are easy to break around heavy iron. It also gives you the look of a newbie weekend warrior. Picture this, you just completed a tough set on the bench press. You grab your phone to harmlessly log your results. At the same time, a veteran iron warrior is fuming because he's waiting on a bench press and it "appears" that you are texting, social media-ing sitting on a bench press! On the flip side, a simple pen and paper workout journal would paint quite a different picture and be much faster. Your image would be instead a fellow iron warrior that takes his training seriously enough to accurately monitor results. The fuming iron warrior will instead be delighted to see a fellow iron warrior who takes his/ her training as serious as they do. They will have instant respect for you. See the difference in perception? Back to rest periods now. Every workout in the *Bradbury Muscle Course* has precisely prescribed rest. It is detailed for you in the training program. The core movements on the strength focus of the workout will have longer rest periods between sets. This is to insure maximal strength on those crucial heavy sets. The isolation movements in the pump focus of the workout will have shorter rest periods. This is to maximize hypertrophy, release favorable hormones, and to achieve a mind-blowing pump every workout. The exact rest period for you to follow for every exercise will be displayed clearly in the *Bradbury Muscle Course*. Make sure to follow the allotted rest periods with precision for maximal results.

Viva La Pump

It is well understood, without a shadow of a doubt, that to maximize muscle growth an extreme pump must be achieved every workout. What exactly is a muscle pump? A muscle pump is a rushing of blood into a muscle being worked. This automatic action is produced by the body when responding to a proper stimulus. The pump literally gorges your muscles with vital nutrients via blood flow. This action amplifies the repair and growth process. The extreme swelling of the muscle also aids in stretching out your fascia around the muscles. Stretching out the fascia allows your muscles to grow even bigger. The feeling of a pump is also very satisfying and a celebratory symbol of a job well done. In an addictive fashion, it is fun to feel and see your muscles blow up to super-human size. Most importantly, all of that swelling is forcing much needed nutrients right where you need it most, directly into your working muscles. The pump usually subsides fairly soon once the training session has ceased. Every workout should achieve a strong muscle pump, especially towards the end of the session. The *Bradbury Muscle Course* is specially designed to make sure this phenomenon occurs every single workout without fail.

HOW TO TAKE YOUR PUMP TO THE NEXT LEVEL:

- Follow the *Bradbury Muscle Course's* prescribed rest periods exactly
- Focus your attention on maintaining muscle tension and squeeze hard every rep
- Get a full stretch and strong contraction of the muscle every rep
- A high quality pre-workout supplement can work wonders
- Stay well hydrated at all times
- Don't get distracted or let your mind wonder, solely focus on the task at hand
- Imagine in your mind literally gorging the muscle with blood during reps
- Follow the *Bradbury Muscle Course* exactly! It is specially designed to deliver a superior pump every workout.

How to Get Crazy Strong

The *Bradbury Muscle Course* is a superior program as it blends only the very best ideas from all styles of training. It has one goal in mind: to build jaw-dropping lean muscle mass that will be the talk of town. As a bonus, this program also draws heavily from the strength training arena. Getting supremely muscular goes hand in hand with getting supremely strong. Like two peas in a pod. In addition to growing an enormous amount of muscle, you will get insanely strong. So this begs the question, how does one go about getting stronger? To be blunt, there are many "tricksters" and "gurus" that hide behind their computer screens with all their "secrets" to superhuman strength. Would you still be interested in all their "secrets" if you knew they were a buck fifty soaking wet and their head sits on top of what appears to be a pixy stick? Naw, I'll pass on those "secrets." They can take their little secrets and shove them up their swiss ball workout. Don't fall victim to these all-to-common scammers. The only reason I wrote this book was to have a way to deliver you RESULTS in a simple format. This is and always will be a results-based program. Frankly, nothing else matters. You do the program and you earn results. The shocking outreach of people desperately searching for answers compelled me. I am utterly appalled at the mass confusion I see among people when it comes to getting visible results. It is completely mind-blowing to be honest. I believe it is a manifestation of years and years of misleading information. I am determined to get in your hands an easy to read and apply program. A program that will deliver what so many truly desire, real tangible results! So many lost souls blindly go around, akin to a merry-go-round, trying new trainers, new programs, the latest fad, a special diet and time after time they go home empty handed. My frustrations grew as I felt much of the industry was built solely on hype and no substance. From day one, I have chased only one thing when helping others and that was to make it my obligation everyday to get them results. Not just any result, but visible, life changing results. My philosophy has always been to keep an open mind, give things a fair shake, and then answer the hardest question of all: DID IT WORK? My mission is to put biases aside and always answer this tough question with brutal honesty to make a sound conclusion. After spending countless hours of intense study, thousands of hours conducting training sessions and learning through trial and error, I have learned and successfully applied how to get people stronger. Most importantly, you get stronger by systematically and correctly applying overload to your body. Most people miss the mark here by making many common rookie mistakes. There is definitely an art to applying progressive overload (see The Art of Progression chapter). Careless and random attempts to add overload is a recipe for disaster. The idea of progressive overload has been around since Milo of Croton carried a calf around everyday until it eventually turned into a bull. In the *Bradbury Muscle Course*, this meticulous work is instructed to the reader and provided in the program. You will learn how to apply the optimal amount of progressive overload for astronomical strength gains over time.

Acquiring strength is not as simple as many people think. Putting more weight on the bar is a major part of getting stronger. However, what if I told you there actually exists 4 different methods of getting stronger? These 4 methods are proven in both the scientific and strength training communities. Would you be interested to learn them now? Most people are left in the dark and succumb to massive frustration and eventual doom with their training program. You, my friend, will be one of the few that has been enlightened and will get to skip all of the frustration.

4 METHODS OF STRENGTH TRAINING:

1. Maximal Effort Method
2. Repeated Effort Method
3. Submaximal Effort Method
4. Dynamic Effort Method

Without boring you to death with a whole bunch of unnecessary details, below is all you need to know to grasp the power that exists in each of these four methods.

MAXIMAL EFFORT METHOD

This is simply an all-out maximum effort with very heavy weight for 1-5 reps. An example would be to work up to a 5 rep max (5RM). This method is solely used on big, compound movements like the bench press or squat. If you are at a beginner level, you should not perform the maximal effort method, rather continue to add weight in a sensible progression. With the maximal effort method, the weights used must be in the range of 85-105% of your 1 rep max. **Think very heavy and low reps!** This method is superior for increasing muscular coordination. It also trains the muscles and central nervous system to be able to exert maximal force. This method is second-to-none for delivering drastic raw strength increases. Although, not the greatest hypertrophy tool, this method should be used in any serious program. The extreme physical and psychological demand of the maximal effort method makes it suitable for only occasional use for our purposes. Doing the Maximal Effort Method too often will quickly lead you to overtraining, frustration and likely injury. Too frequent use of this method is a disaster waiting to happen. We will implement the maximal effort method at the proper time in the *Bradbury Muscle Course*. I repeat, if you are a beginner, make sure you master the movements and gain much experience before embarking on this method. If you are a beginner and the program calls for a maximal effort (work up and establish a 1-5 rep max) just make a smart, sensible jump. Let's say you completed 5 reps on the bench press with 150lbs last time and now the current week calls for to work up to a 1-5RM. You will simply perform 5 reps with 152-155lbs, a sensible jump, and call it a day on that movement. You earned progress and got stronger. Do not, by any circumstance, be a fool and try to keep forcing heavier and heavier weights when you are a newbie. You will never grow muscle if you are injured all the time. Train smart!

REPEATED EFFORT METHOD

In this method, you will be using a non-maximal weight and performing reps until complete failure. When we say failure, it means absolute failure. If you do not completely reach failure, you are not doing the repeated effort method properly. During the crucial last few reps of the grueling set your muscles will have to produce a max force to lift the weight, despite being in a highly fatigued state. Your muscles will be on fire the last couple reps! I love this method, because it is truly a muscle and strength builder. In addition to building slabs of muscle, this method recruits an extremely high amount of all muscle fiber types. A moderate weight should be used for usually 8-30 reps. You will continue to perform reps with good form until complete failure. This method must be precisely administered and not be overused as it will surely tend to make you slip into overtraining rather quickly. Sets for this method will read: 3 x MAX REPS. I love to use bodyweight movements on this like dips. Make sure to always have competent spotters and/or utilize a commercial-grade power rack with sturdy pins to catch weight if applicable.

SUBMAXIMAL EFFORT METHOD

This method makes up the bulk of any serious muscle hypertrophy program. This is the king kong method of our program! This method is just like the repeated effort method except for one important difference. You use non-maximal weights, but you do not go until complete failure. This is a superior muscle builder and presents a very low chance for injury and can be done frequently. This is what we call a win-win! The majority of reps ranges will fall between 5-15 reps to maximize muscle hypertrophy. This method helps to activate a boatload of motor units and muscle fibers. The main goal of this method is to spark muscle growth, a perfect solution for our purposes. In addition, this method also helps to improve strength.

DYNAMIC EFFORT METHOD

The Dynamic Effort Method (D.E. Method) is to be used with lighter weights of 50-80% of your 1 rep max. Generally, this is done with low reps (2-3) with an emphasis on moving the bar as fast as possible on the way up. You will attempt to put as much force as possible into the barbell in hopes of increasing bar speed. The goal of this method is to increase the rate of force development. This means to condition your body to blast through neuro-inhibitors to produce a maximal force as fast as possible. The *Bradbury Muscle Course* being a focused muscle growth program uses this method sparingly as it has a poor hypertrophy response versus other methods.

However, we do use it occasionally in the program with explosive push presses and squats to ramp up full body power. The dynamic method is well known to help powerlifters blast through sticking points and lift more explosively. Generally, it will be displayed with a higher number of sets and with 2-3 reps with very short rest periods. (Example: D.E. Back Squat 8x2; 30 seconds rest)

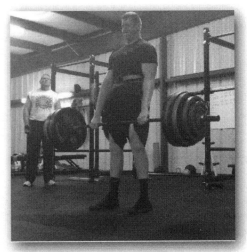

No worries, you'll be as strong as you look!

Although the *Bradbury Muscle Course's* main focus is on growing muscle, it also provides a very potent strength training stimulus. It systematically implements all 4 of the strength methods discussed above. This will put you lightyears ahead of many of the "strength only" programs out there. This gives you the best of both worlds! Shocking strength levels and at the same time stunning muscularity.

19

The Art of Progression

This might be the most important lesson to learn so pay very close attention and take notes! Have you ever attempted to get a suntan? Getting a nice tan in time for lake season is a pretty simple task if done correctly. However, done wrong it can turn into a hellish nightmare. Imagine, you decide you want a tan and you take your pasty self outside and tough out 4 hours in the beating summer sun. Not only will people soon mistake you as a giant mutated lobster walking around, but you may have a trip to the hospital in your near future. Sadly, misguided people take this insane route with their training all too often. The deceptive lure of instant gratification and the foolish "more is better" attitude gobbles up many victims. Now, just think if that same person had just gone out for just 10 minutes in the sun. A couple days later, they went out again for 12 minutes. Then a few days later, they go out for 15 minutes and so on and so forth making sensible increases in exposure without ever overdoing it. Painlessly, they would achieve a wonderful beach ready tan in just a matter of weeks.

Your body adapts much the same way when it comes to proper training. A very small progress every training session will take you a long way over time. One of the biggest mistakes I see plaguing overzealous lifters is trying to make too big of increases in load or reps. Instead, make friends with the small plates to end up with the big boys one day. You must trust and embrace the process. The 5lb, 2.5lb, and even 1lb plates should see playing time every training session. If for some odd reason your gym doesn't have 1lb plates bring your own. You can buy or make some for a few dollars. Let's say for example you have completed week 1 and you completed 10 reps with 200lbs on the bench press. Then on week 3 when you tackle this workout again, the wise man would add 2-5lbs. This would make it 202-205lbs for a set of 10, a very sensible progression. Always take the progress, no matter how small it is. Progress always tastes better than failure. Trust me, you will have plenty of time to add more weight down the road. It's good to be ambitious, but greed is always a fool's game. The fatal flaw is to get greedy and add too much weight too soon just to quickly get stuck in a frustrating plateau. The *Bradbury Muscle Course* is specially designed to keep you feeling strong and fresh at all times. Every time you tackle the full 12-week *Bradbury Muscle Course* cycle you will see improvements with your weights lifted and visibly on your physique. This will help you stay highly motivated to keep on trucking. Your mental fuel will be seeing your enormous new muscle and strength gains. I see no reason to get stuck in a plateau for a very long time with this program if you check your ego at the door and make smart jumps in weight. With the revolutionary design of the *Bradbury Muscle Course*, you have the perfect training program that you will reap results from for years to come.

3 WEEK PHASE 1 PROGRESSION EXAMPLE:

Bench Press

Week 1: 135x10

Week 2: Incline Bench Press 5x10

Week 3: 140x10

20

Grow with Growth Weeks

There is no denying that the key to getting results is working at a high intensity. The act of growing muscle is no different. You must work very hard, but you must be smart. Although a self-sacrificial attitude can be admirable, a severe level of excessive stress on your body will often lead to dismal results and severe consequences. Remember, no matter what you must always pay the fiddler. Too many times enthusiastic trainees fall victim to the idiotic "more is better" approach. This always has a sour ending. You'll be sure to overtax your system and cause short and long term irreversible damage to your body. You will also cause your training to become stale and an undesirable chore. Your muscles will go flat and strength will plummet. Your intensity will also plummet due to a total lack of motivation and interest. Lastly, this "more is better" ideology often leads to an instant severe injury or worse a long-term repetitive use injury that can be career ending. Don't be hardheaded and become your own worse enemy! I don't know about you, but I love to lift weights and grow muscle. The feeling of building your body up is unexplainable. It just feels good to feel good! You want to be able to continue to do what you love dearly well into your golden years. There is a better way. Our program is designed to keep you feeling fresh and strong at all times. Gone are the days of extreme CNS fatigue and feeling beat up all the time. I've found if you feel great everyday it will lead to much more productive workouts, more dynamic results, and without the frustration from a lack of progress.

A major factor to help insure this happens is what I like to call Growth Weeks. These are periodically scheduled in the *Bradbury Muscle Course*. In case you did not know, your muscles don't actually grow during workouts. The workouts serve as a stimulus in which the body must respond. This precise amount of stimulus is then reacted to by the body. If full recovery is achieved, the body supercompensates by becoming a bigger and stronger version of itself. This is to make sure you are ready and prepared for the next onslaught of training. This is considered recovery and muscles grow during this period. One thing I have noticed in my own training and the training of others is that after 3 weeks of intense training your intensity and strength begins to fade off into the sunset like a cowboy at the end of a western film. You'll start to notice feeling stale and won't have the vigor needed to keep training at a high enough intensity to drive adaptations. Our solution: Growth Weeks. Growth Weeks are utilized in our program on weeks 4, 8, and 12. A Growth Week is simply a week of training with lower volume and lower intensity. This allows any accumulated fatigue to diminish out of your body. This also provides your tendons and ligaments time to fully heal up and get stronger. Most importantly, it provides an ample amount of time to let your muscles to fully recover and grow! Your muscles will become bigger and more dense following a Growth Week. This means your body is fully supercompensated from the intense three weeks of training prior to the Growth

Week. You will be shocked at your refreshed mind and deep desire to get back to pushing heavy iron again. This motivation surge will keep your intensity very high to continue to reap great results. This technique will also help tremendously to keep your body in a healthy state. Your tendons and ligaments will thank you for allowing them to also fully recover and adapt. Undoubtably, Growth Weeks will help to minimize your risk of injury. If you choose to utilize a caffeinated pre-workout supplement, it is a great idea to cease use of it during growth weeks. Your body is amazing in it's ability to adapt to any stimulus including your pre-workout drink. By laying off of the pre-workout supplements for a week it will help to diminish your tolerance and help to make the pre-workout supplements work even better once you return to normal intensity. The weights and volume are significantly less during the Growth Week so you won't need the extra boost from a pre-workout, so no worries. Growth Weeks are a perfect time to hone in your technique on your movements since the weights are relatively light. You can get laser focused on moving better and feeling the muscles working during this week. The mission of this week is to give your body a break and let it fully heal and grow. If you are feeling sore and tired after the Growth Week you are doing it completely wrong and most likely not following the program. The *Bradbury Muscle Course* will lay out exactly what to do. The workouts on these crucial weeks are short and easy. This is active recovery at it's finest. Don't be a goofball and screw it up by adding stuff. If you must be an over-achiever and do extra stuff, do some extra foam rolling and light mobility work.

21

"One Top Set" Versus "Sets Across"

The question of should you do sets across or one top set has been hotly debated for years. Sets across means using the same weight across all work sets. For example, sets across would be 5 sets of 10 reps using 200lbs every set. In contrast, one top set would look like 5 sets of 10 reps completed with the first set at 175lbs, the second set with 195bs, and the third set with 205lbs. The fourth set with 210lbs, and then the fifth set with 185lbs. As you can see there is a top set climaxing at 210lbs. Here is a simpler way to look at it as if it were written in your workout log.

Sets Across: Bench Press 5x10 200-200-200-200-200

One Top Set: Bench Press 5x10 175-195-205-210*-185   (*top set)

To start off the comparison, both of these methods have merit. Both will make you stronger. I think it really boils down to how you're wired up mentally and physically. It also depends on your training level. Some people thrive with the sets across and others find them boring as hell, myself included. The sets across is a surefire way to go if you are a rank beginner. Since your work weights are lower than someone who has been in the iron game for years. A beginner can afford the extra practice with a load that will cause adaptations. However, if you have gotten strong most times you will find sets across excruciatingly demanding both mentally and physically. Compare 5 sets of 5 with a 185lb squat versus 5 sets of 5 with a 550lb squat. Yikes! Being able to complete 5 sets across with 550lbs on your back would take quite the toll. So here is my verdict. I am not saying I am right and others are wrong, because I have trained both ways and know they both work. I am just telling you from experience what works better for me and in the observation of training others. Unless you are a beginner, I think that sets across on the heavy stuff becomes extremely taxing mentally and physically as you become stronger and stronger. With sets across people tend to rush warm-up sets to get to the goal weight and then grind out the reps and sets with the same weight. I also find sets across a little on the boring side. From my training and the training of others, I feel that people lift more explosively when it counts with one top set. I believe your body is designed to take on more and more weight gradually building up to your potential best set for that day. Your body is more geared up and ready for the work at hand because of the mindset that you only have to do the heaviest set once. Common sense tells us that lifting explosively is better than lifting with a grinding, slow pace. One top set seems to align well with this theory. With one top set, you will be able to use more weight for one set which will spark adaptation. If you've ever lifted weights before, you'd agree it just feels right to go up a little bit each set and then muster up all the strength you've got and blast through an almighty top set. Make sure to log all work sets in your training log and especially the top set. Then move on to the next exercise celebrating your victory of getting stronger. Another way to make up for volume is to utilize a back off set or two. A back off set is simply using less weight than your top set to finish out the prescribed sets. For example, say you are supposed to do 295lbs for 5 reps on bench press this week. A well executed one top set scheme with a back off set would look something like this (not including lighter warm-up sets):

TOP SET WITH A BACK-OFF SET
265x5
275x5
285x5
295x5*GOAL
275x5

TOP SET WITHOUT A BACK-OFF SET
255x5
265x5
275x5
285x5
295x5*GOAL

As you can imagine there are literally thousands of different ways to work up to a one top set successfully. As long as you are seeing your top set increasing in weight from cycle to cycle you are on the right track. The best way to figure out how to make proper jumps set to set is through trial and error. Experience is your best teacher. Some people like to make bigger jumps and others like smaller jumps. Some like to reach their goal weight sooner and others like to go for it on the very last set. Now that we have covered how to structure your sets in the strength focus portions of the workouts now we need to cover something of extreme importance. Please recall the sensible jumps and suntan in the art of progression chapter. For this program to work long term you must stick to the plan! You will get much more muscular and stronger in the long run if you will stay disciplined. Rigid, unwavering discipline will always keep you on the right track. Do not become foolish and derail yourself. If you are a beginner make jumps of 5-10lbs religiously. You can't go wrong with 5lb jumps and that is what I would recommend for a beginner. As you put more skin in the game and get stronger you will be looking at 2-5lb jumps and even smaller if needed. To make this very clear here is a 3 week plan that aligns with our program for a beginner:

SQUAT 5X5 WITH ONE TOP SET:
Week 1: 105,125,145,155,135
Week 2: Front Squat 5x5
Week 3: 110,130,150,160,140

Always stick to your plan. Only a fool would get caught up in the moment and make too big of jumps and get stuck. This mistake happens all to often. You have been warned. Earning as much muscle as possible is a marathon and not a sprint. Trust the process. Remember, nobody built show stopping biceps laying on a surgeon's table. Alway train smart! You are smart because you have this book and you are set up to win and win big. Do not let anything or anybody derail you from guaranteed results.

Magic of 11'S

Many will ask, "what's with the 11 reps?" You will notice that on the "pump focus" section the frequent use of sets of 11 reps. The reason being that the smack dab middle of the hypertrophy rep range is 11.5. The range of 8-15 reps has been tested and proven in the fancy labs of academia and in the trenches of dusty hardcore gyms for years. This rep range reigns superior for growing muscle by provoking maximal hypertrophy. The precise middle between 8-15 is 11.5. Oddly, since all sets start with the number one, I find it much easier to count to 11 being an odd number versus 10 or 12. Maybe it's just how my brain is wired, but I'd bet when you start doing 11's you will experience this too. Eleven reps also gives you a cushion on both sides to maximize return even if you make an error counting or choosing a weight. Have you ever lost count and did one or two extra reps to make sure you covered the prescribed number? Have, perhaps, your eyes been bigger than your muscles and you used too much weight and came up a few reps short? With 11's there is no harm, no foul because you will still fall into the 8-15 range even if you make a mistake. However, if you are prescribed a set of 8 and you make the same mistake of taking too much weight you will unfortunately fall out of the hypertrophy range. Potential muscle growth is lost to another day. Do the 11's the *Bradbury Muscle Course* prescribes and I know you will notice a difference as you'll see your muscles respond by growing and keep growing. Scrawny skeptics will argue, "oh, there is not that much difference between doing 11's verses 10's or 12's!" They may be right, but try it and see for yourself. I've enjoyed less counting errors and optimal muscle growth from 11's and you will too. It's just like how some people like their steaks well-done, medium, and of course rare and bloody. Everyone is wired up different. Elevens put you in the best possible scenario to root your training into the heart of the hypertrophy range. It is a simple hack that is fool proof, sets you up to win every set and it works! It takes doing the uncommon to avoid being common.

Crush the Bar!

Let's do a quick test:

1. Flex your bicep with your hand open as hard as you can for 5 seconds
2. Shake out your arm
3. Make and maintain a super tight fist and flex the same bicep again for 5 seconds
4. Feel the difference!

When you did the little test above you could feel the big difference the second time you flexed your bicep with a tight fist. Your bicep flexed harder and you can feel all the other forearm muscles working in sync to deliver a much more intense contraction. This simple 15 second test is a strong lesson to learn for when you lift weights. Always no matter what CRUSH THE BAR! This simple technique can mean the difference in drastically improving your bench press or not. It can save your elbows from nagging pain that could manifest and bring a halt to your training. Personally, I envision my fingers putting dents into the bar or dumbbell every single rep without fail. Aesthetically speaking, your forearms will grow like weeds if you utilize this technique every time you train. Mark my words, you will never see an impressive bench presser with snowman twigs hanging off their elbows. Another added bonus, if you are a single dude looking to land that first date, studies have shown that one of the first body parts women notice on men is their forearms. In the business world, nothing speaks louder than a great first impression finished off with a solid, firm handshake. All the more reason to crush the bar! You can thank me later when you land that home run career and marry the girl of your dreams.

How to Warm Up

Did you know that most devastating injuries could have been easily been prevented by a proper warm up? A good 7-8 minute warm-up or a ruptured quad? It's your choice. I think I'll go with the proper warm up every time. Nothing can make you injury proof, but a great warm-up greatly reduces the risk of injury. Now there are literally thousands of ways to warm up. You can find articles written by these 135lb "gurus" bashing all kinds of different warm up protocols and movements. Don't waste your time or energy! This book in your hands gives you all you need to know. You master this book and you master how to build muscle. Truly it is that simple. As for proper warm ups, I have 3 principles that will always put your body in a primed state to maximize performance and safety. Follow these principles and your body will be ready to demolish your workout. If you don't adhere to all of these principles you will hit the weights feeling flat and wimpy.

3 PRINCIPLES:

1. Raise Core Body Temperature
2. Establish Range of Motion
3. Perform Specific Movement Lightly

Let's go over each of these so there is zero confusion on how to execute the 3 principles. Let's say today is an upper body workout leading off with the incline bench press. To raise your core body temperature you will do 5 minutes on a rower machine, arm cycle or an air bike. I'd recommend some movement that involves your upper body for the 5 minutes. This gets your body temperature up, blood flowing and heart thumping. Psychologically, it makes you ready to hit the iron. It builds the rage and many times you will start to feel aggressive during your warm up. You'll be getting primed to absolutely attack the weights. This is far superior than hitting your 1st set with flat muscles that are colder than a witch's tit in a brass bra. After 5 minutes, you will now work to establish a full range of motion. For this example, I'd recommend use a softball to roll out pecs and do some light rows to get your chest moving in full range. Dynamic stretching is superior for warm ups. Therefore, arm circles and extremely light chest flys will help to bring about full range of motion and start to pump blood into the area about to be worked. Now for the final phase of warm up it is time to get specific! Our first exercise is incline bench press. So, we warm up with light leg press? No dummy! Don't make this complicated. We start with incline bench presses with an empty bar. Personally, I like to do 20 reps slow and methodical and then follow up with 15 reps slow and methodical. Both sets are with an empty bar or very light weight. Believe it or not, nobody has ever won a gold medal in warm-ups. Now you should be in the groove of the movement with full range of motion. Blood should be rushing the area. You should also start to feel the euphoria of feeling primed to pump iron. Lastly, work up to your work set weight with multiple build up sets. Say your first work set of 10 is with 165lbs. You will want to do some reps with 95lbs, 125lbs, 145lbs before hitting that first work set. Your body is designed to be prepared for intense work in this manner. Always follow these principles without fail! This will lead you to much safer and productive training sessions. Remember, an once of prevention is worth a pound of cure. If you are in a time crunch, do not be an idiot and skip the warm up and injure yourself. It would be a better outcome to do the warm up and half the workout versus rushing into it just to get to set up an appointment with an orthopedic surgeon the next day. A word of wisdom, if you ever find yourself feeling rushed into or during a workout, WATCH OUT! Extreme danger is lurking right around the corner. Take your time and let your body charge up like it is meant to do. Your performance will skyrocket! The example given is specific for a workout leading off with an incline bench press. As you can see you can easily apply these 3 principles to any workout.

Workout Log

A simple workout log can be the difference between success and failure. I am a pen and paper guy. I do not like using a phone. Between you and me phones in the gym get on my nerves. Pen and paper is faster, cheaper and looks cooler when you have stacks of old workout logs sitting in your library. "Look kiddos this is the first time grandpa deadlifted 600 when I was a young whipper snapper and back then we had to walk to the gym 5 miles uphill both ways in 3 feet of snow." -grandpa iron warrior. Pen and paper are timeless. Think of all the awesome photos and information that can be lost instantly when a phone falls into the bottom of a lake. I'm skeptical and don't trust that "cloud" thingy either. What if you had 2 decades of training logged on the "cloud" and it decided to rain and the "cloud" suddenly disappeared? Perception of phones is whack too. Picture yourself sitting on a bench press, in a crowded gym, harmlessly logging your workout on your phone. However, everyone's perception is that you are playing on social media, posing for a gym selfie, or texting. This is not how to win friends. Phones are a huge distraction for you and others. You are crushing your workout in a extremely focused manner and then out of nowhere you get an angry text message from someone all upset with you. All of sudden your mind wanders and you might as well just go home, because nothing good will come from an unfocused workout. Leave your phone in the car or better yet throw it into the trashcan. Instead, invest a few dollars into a workout log. I prefer the kind that are specifically designed to log strength training workouts. Many people do fine with a simple composition book or notebook. Find whichever works best for you. Then you get yourself a nice pen or pencil. Instead of having to open apps and making typos you can jot down your results extremely fast using pen and paper. This is truly revolutionary stuff. I like to log everything. However, it is a MUST to log the "strength focus" part of your workouts. Many will find the "pump focus" weights to go with how you are feeling that day. Which is fine, this can be considered using the instinctive principle. The "strength focus" portion must be tracked to know how much weight to add next session and to measure long term progress. Make sure to record your sets, reps, weight used and your bodyweight every week. Also, note how you are feeling that day as well just for reference reasons. The *Bradbury Muscle Course* is designed to make sure you always feel fresh and ready to attack. You do have to live life and maybe you got only 2 hours of sleep last night. We all know this will affect training so just make a quick note of it. The *Bradbury Muscle Course* is the last program you will ever need to grow muscle now and to keep growing forever. Make sure to write everything down. It is delightfully motivating to scan back several months of training cycles to see the measurable progress you've experienced. As mentioned earlier this program is for maximal muscle growth, but you will also enjoy enormous strength gains. So get your pen and notebook ready to record your gains!

The Ten Commandments of Muscle

These must never be broken for everlasting growth!

1) **Thou Shall Stay The Path** - Many times people will get into working out and once the newness wears off they ride off into the sunset like the ending of a western film. This is usually due to faulty program design that leads to frustration. You have the best program that will grow muscle and keep you highly motivated at all times. Too much variety and the results are sparse. Too little variety and training becomes mundane, enthusiasm is non-existent and intensity goes down the toilet. All of these potential pitfalls are taken care of in the *Bradbury Muscle Course*. You have just enough variety to never become stale and the perfect blend to keep the visible results coming. Seeing great results for your efforts fuels even more motivation and this turns into a vicious cycle. After reading this book, you should understand the true power of this program and should never stray. At all costs stay the path. Make the needed adjustments in your life to make sure you can get your training sessions in and always strive to keep your diet susceptible to gaining lean muscle, but not fat.

2) **Thou Shall Not Be Betrayed By False Data** - Millions of articles surface the internet, magazines, etc. Their #1 goal is to grab your attention and get you to click on it or buy a magazine or product. This is all about, you guessed it, money. Cha-ching! Most of the time your results aren't even on their radar. They just want to entice you enough to take action by clicking or buying while they make money on the back-end by selling ads. Don't fall for this junk. Especially, do not start trying to mash the latest "super secret technique" into the *Bradbury Muscle Course*. This program works way too well to get mashed up with other training "philosophies." Follow the program exactly and you will be astonished at the results. The cool thing is that it actually works and at the highest level possible. Many of the "gurus" out there hide behind their keyboards and computer screens and they have no clue what really works. Don't be foolish. Follow this program and none others. Give it at least 1 year and the results will be superhuman. Just imagine if you followed it for 5 years straight.

3) **Thou Shall Stay Hydrated** - Did you know that your muscles are made up of over 70% water? Being dehydrated will wreck havoc on your training. Your muscle pump will be lousy. Strength levels will plummet. Even your protein synthesis will be derailed while living in a dehydrated state. Your muscle breakdown rate will skyrocket when you are dehydrated. Even being slightly dehydrated will still cause major problems. Being dehydrated can even lead to severe and chronic depression since your brain tissue is

over 80% water. I'm not about to put on a lab coat and start making a thousand different recommendations and crazy formulas of how much water to drink and when. You should know by now that I always keep it simple. If your urine is the color of root beer go to the hospital immediately. If your urine is a dark yellow you need to drink more water. If your urine is a very light yellow you are right on track and keep doing what you are doing. If your urine is completely clear you can back off just a touch. Adhere to this commandment at all costs. You will enjoy a more positive outlook and a happier life. You will feel better and have more energy. You will get sick less often. Most importantly, you'll have bigger muscles.

4) **Thou Shall Become Strong** - The guiding principle of this program is bigger is stronger, stronger is bigger. A major portion of the *Bradbury Muscle Course* is focused on getting stronger. Take all the fancy powerlifting suits away and a man with a 400lb bench press will have a more impressive upper body than a man with a 160lb bench press every single time. This is just the way it is. Always has been and always will be. Our program dedicates a "strength focus" portion of every workout. It's dedicated to make you stronger year after year without fail. Attack every workout with the ambition to get stronger. Part of earning more muscle is getting stronger. Embrace the wonderful sound of 45's clanking together as this will be music to your ears every training day. Take pride in acquiring superhuman strength.

5) **Thou Shall Be Precise With Calories** - If you want to grow muscle, you must eat calories in a surplus. If you need to shed extra body fat you must be in a caloric deficiency. You will learn all the details of how to gain or lose weight at will in the nutrition section. However, if you are a skinny dude make sure to eat plenty of calories. Ideally, the majority of these calories will come from nutrient-dense food sources. To add muscle to your frame you must be in a calorie surplus. If you are in a calorie deficient and lacking sufficient amino acids, please understand your body loves to cannibalize your hard earned muscle mass for fuel. It makes zero sense to work hard in the gym, but flunk out by not eating precisely and correctly. Many skinny guys go around telling people that they "eat a ton" and in reality they eat under 2000 calories a day. Yet they wonder why their biceps rival a twelve year old schoolboy. It's a great idea to get a calorie counter book or app and carefully track your caloric consumption for a few weeks. This will show you exactly how many calories you are actually eating. Many are shocked to find out they are completely missing the mark and they have falsely believed they have been eating enough. When in fact their lack of muscle was a direct reflection of their puny diet. Always aim to eat enough calories to support activities and muscle growth, but be cautious not to eat too many to accumulate excess fat.

6) **Thou Shall Never Make Excuses** - You think you have it tough, but you don't. There have been numerous physique superstars that have worked grueling hours at highly demanding jobs too. There have been people who's genetics have given them a bad draw, but they countered by playing the proper hand. They took lemons and made lemonade. Everyone puts their pants on one leg at a time. Do not get caught up in the misinformation and start blaming your parents, gym, muscle insertions, <insert whiny excuse here>, etc. Anyone equipped with the *Bradbury Muscle Course* will build a commanding physique that will be admired by others. Truly, in time, you will become a show-stopper! You will never make it happen if you sit around wasting energy making excuses. It's too hot, It's too cold, I'm tired, I'm sick, I don't feel strong today, the weights feel heavy, I'm too sore, my gym is too small, my gym is too big, my workout

partner is lame, etc etc etc. Would you like me to continue? I'm sure not. One thing that all chronic excuse-makers have in common is that nobody can stand to be around them. Don't join the ranks of the unlikable. Remember, if you walk with the lame you will develop a limp. Stay away from chronic excuse-makers at all costs as they will drag you into the deep depths of misery. Misery loves company. Excuses never built any muscle and never will. Avoid excuses like the plague!

7) ***Thou Shall Believe In Yourself*** - Belief is an extremely powerful tool. I will take the guy with less talent that believes in himself over the guy with tons of talent with a doubtful attitude any day of the week. You gotta believe! Believe that you will have 18+" arms. Believe that your current bench max will become easy warm ups one day. I'm here to tell you that if you believe in yourself and believe in this program the result will be nothing short of remarkable. No one becomes an uncommon achiever if they are a doubting Thomas. Jump in with both feet, because those are the guys who make all the progress. The goober sitting on the sideline frozen in time by analysis paralysis doesn't make anything happen. If you are into analytics and doing math problems go for it, but come with me if you want to build muscle and lots of it. You might as well believe in yourself, because nobody else will until you do. If you told ten of your best friends that you are going to have a 50+ inch chest by this time next year, do you think they'd all believe you? Probably not. However, if you believed it and achieved it and then showed them with a tape measurer in hand they would all become instant believers. Seeing is believing! However, the life-changing results are only reserved for the people who believe it before they can see it.

8) ***Thou Shall Find Rest*** - Like the Yin Yang, optimal muscle growth must be obtained through a delicate balance of stimulation and recovery. Too little of either one and your results will suffer. A large part of the recovery system of the human body is proper sleep. You must get plenty of sound sleep. Good sleep patterns lead to a better mood, more energy, less ugly fat and more muscle. You must get at least 8 full hours of sleep. Many average people can sleep a lot less, however, they are average. You are looking to grow muscle and build strength. You put hard work into your career and into your training. It only makes sense that you need more recovery to balance out the higher amounts stimulation than the average couch potato. You make your training (stimulation) a priority so you must also make your recovery a priority. You can also enhance recovery by utilizing naps during the day. Going outside and sitting peacefully in nature for 30 minutes 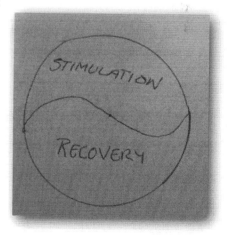 can do wonders for your body. Naps and nature meditation will help you fully relax, release tensions and can facilitate recovery. Exquisite photo drawn by yours truly.

9) ***Thou Shall Slash Stressors*** - As mentioned above, hardcore training is a strong stimulation to your body. Intense workouts produce a high level of stress. Couple that with common stressors related to work, school, kids, people, etc and you can amass a lot of accumulative stress. While on your muscle building quest, you must try to minimize any and all extra stressors. If there are certain people who cause you great stress you must avoid them. If you add stress to your body by drinking excessive alcohol or

smoking cigarettes you must eliminate those habits. You must banish any avoidable stressors! If you like to pound donuts and funnel cakes on Saturday night, STOP! If you have an allergic reaction from mowing the grass, go buy a pack of allergen reducing face masks. If you want the most muscle growth possible, minimize any physical activity outside of the *Bradbury Muscle Course*. If a buddy wants you to go hiking up a mountain somewhere kindly decline and stay home to recover. Always remember that any physical activity adds more stress to which you must recover from. That means more stress to combat and less muscle growth. Excessive stress levels lead to a nasty hormone release (cortisol) that ravages lean muscle tissue and packs on ugly fat. It is fashionable, at the time of the writing of this book, to wear these little bracelets that are supposed to tell you how "fit" you supposedly are by walking countless steps and prancing around. Personally, I do not wear one of these devices and dislike how they reward aimless activities and for the most part disregard the lifting of heavy iron. Even though it's proven that resistance training is responsible for all muscular transformations. If you are more concerned about your boy-scout conditioning level than building muscle, this program may not be your cup of tea. Go download a couch to 5k or something. No hard feelings. If you train with the *Bradbury Muscle Course* and abide by the prescribed rest periods you will build exceptional conditioning along with your newly acquired muscle. Always remember that random exercise leads to random results. On the contrary, specialized training leads to focused results. Which brings us to our 10th and final commandment of muscle…

10) ***Thou Shall Specialize*** - This shouldn't come as a surprise to anyone, but if you want something you must focus on it. The opposite would be some poor, misguided soul falsely believing that if they play countless hours of baseball they will be able to one day enjoy a career in professional hockey. You know and I know that this approach is a sure-fire way to failure. Another fashionable approach would be to play a little baseball, golf, tennis, football, ping pong and water polo to become a professional hockey player. Again, this approach will only give you only dismal results toward your ultimate goal. You must focus on what you want through specialization. There is no other way. If you want muscle, you must specialize in building muscle. Sure any shyster could write a very convincing sales pitch claiming that the secret to build 18+ inch arms, drug-free, is to run a marathon. Unfortunately, some people would believe the hype, jump on board and blindly follow this utterly wrong advice. However, a wise man would know this would not work and that route would actually put you even further from your goal of 18+ inch arms. Make sure your training aligns precisely with your goal. If you want to build lots of muscle then the *Bradbury Muscle Course* is second-to-none as it specializes solely on growing muscle. If your goal is to complete an ultra-marathon this program is not the program for you as it only specializes in building maximal amounts of muscle. It does not specialize in running over 26.2 miles without stopping. To receive the results you want you must enter the proper commands. As mentioned before, it is just like the old DOS computers. If you accidentally enter an incorrect command by mistyping a single letter or punctuation, the computer cannot do anything with it. It shoots it back as a user error. However, if you enter the command perfectly the computer delivers the function you desired immediately. Your body is the same way. Sadly, a great number of people spend hours and countless dollars entering the wrong command over and over again. They never receive the results they so deeply desire. They work extremely hard, pour gallons of sweat, huff and

puff, but never get the visible results they are chasing after. Just like a dog chasing it's tail. Most of the time this is due to the workout program they are following just isn't giving the body the proper command and thus it computes a user error and rejects the input. This is why you must specialize and always give your body the proper command! By giving your body the right command you are on the superhighway to the results you want. If muscle mass and razor-sharp definition is what you are seeking, the *Bradbury Muscle Course* will deliver the precise commands into your body and you will see the difference.

27

The Forgotten Show Muscles

To put it bluntly, this chapter is about how to look jacked in street clothes. Many programs neglect the all-important "show" muscles. Let's get something clear, with this program all of your muscles will be put into the optimal position to grow to their maximal potential. You will notice a major visible difference after the first 12-week cycle of the *Bradbury Muscle Course*. It is appalling after reviewing hundreds of different programs, many have a common glaring absence. The most visible muscles have been completely abandoned! It is common knowledge that the neck, forearms and calves are the most visible muscles in street clothes. Our program doesn't make this rookie mistake and we attack them with a vengeance. Your commanding physique will get noticed even in the loosest of street clothes. Gone are the days of the awkward smedium t-shirts.

Forearms - You will never meet a truly strong man with fragile forearms. The ability to powerfully grasp an object or person is essential. Whether you are defending yourself or hanging onto your new deadlift PR. Your forearm strength will either make you or break you. I shouldn't fail to mention that if you are a single guy looking to attract a spouse that studies have shown that women take notice of forearms before numerous other body parts. They are a true symbol of dominance and are highly visible in any short sleeve shirt. People, when they meet you, will undoubtably see your bulging forearms and will consciously and subconsciously recognize supreme power and will treat you with the upmost respect. A strong, firm handshake always reigns supreme over the dreaded "dead fish" handshake. The *Bradbury Muscle Course* utilizes an arsenal of movements that will give you the ultimate forearm development. From hanging on to heavy iron to special exercises that will develop your forearms to their maximum potential. Most notably, the Zottman Curl is a staple throughout the program. This old school arm builder is rightly named after a 19th century strongman George Zottman. The unique twisting pattern stimulates virtually every muscle in your arm. It is also one of the finest bicep builders out there.

Neck - Unless you are in a Ghillie suit about to go hunting, your neck is most likely visible to the public. Nothing screams sheer strength and athleticism like big traps and a muscular neck. When people see your traps bulging out of the back of your shirt they'll know not to try to push you around. Your neck strength is vital to survival and could potentially save your life. If you've ever seen an elite football player you'll notice that they will have a bigger neck than say a basketball player. This is simply because they depend on their neck muscles to sustain the position of their spine during blows to the head. If you've got a pencil neck and take a serious shot to the head it can mean terrible news. I am going to be a little blunt here so prepare yourself. If you take a look around at our general population most people's posture just plain sucks! This is great news if you are a chiropractor, but not if you are looking to hoist the big weights and grow lots of muscle any time soon. Big, strong traps, upper back and neck essentially cure a bad posture. Years of desk work and slumped sitting can be virtually undone in just matter of weeks with our program. Our main trap builders are a steady dose of regular shrugs, deadlifts, farmer's walk and one of my all-time favorites the power shrug. In addition to packing slabs of muscle onto your frame and developing explosive full body power, the power shrug is a serious neck and trap builder. This game changing exercise coupled with plenty of regular shrugs and you will be stretching out your shirt collars in no time.

Calves - Anytime you decide to wear shorts your calves are going to show. Some people are born with a great set of calves and others are not. Both cases should work them to reach their maximum potential. The lucky few with already large calves will work to further chisel and define them. People born with less than stellar calves will have to work them hard and often! Calves are stubborn muscles with loads of endurance. Even if you've had tough draw, you can still play the hand to maximize your potential. Say you got scrawny calves with super high insertions from your parents, you can still grow your calves to a very respectable level through hard work. Although, it's true that your calves will grow from heavy squats, deadlifts, etc. Like any muscle, to achieve optimal development you must focus and apply direct work through isolation movements. On the following page, is one of the toughest calf building protocols you'll ever do. I call it the Calf Blast. This supplementary calf routine will grow anyone's calves and it only takes a few minutes to complete. If calves are a weakness for you, feel free to do a few extra calf blasts in addition to what the *Bradbury Muscle Course* calls for. You can tackle this 2-5 times per week. However, I would recommend to start out really light and work your way up in a sensible fashion to avoid a crippling overuse injury. All you need is a 2"x4" and a dip belt. You can also use a standing or seated calf machine. Personally, I prefer the dip belt loaded with plates to minimize compressive forces on your spine. When you do the repetition burnout portion you will perform these reps quickly, but not wildly out of control. You will continue for as many reps as possible until you cannot move your heel even an inch. Don't worry about counting the reps on the burnout, just try to think of things to take your mind off the intense burn. Enjoy this gut buster and watch your calves grow like weeds in the spring!

Calf Blast

Use same weight throughout

Perform 15 reps (slow and controlled)

Rest 10 seconds (shake out legs)

Perform 12 reps (slow and controlled)

Rest 10 seconds (shake out legs)

Perform 10 reps (slow and controlled)

Rest 10 seconds (shake out legs)

Perform a repetition burnout (until you cannot move your heal 1")

Rest 10 seconds (shake out legs)

Perform 10 single leg eccentric reps (go slow as possible)

Rest 10 seconds (shake out legs)

Perform a repetition burnout (until you cannot move your heel 1")

Stretch out calves

28

How to Lose Fat and Gain Muscle at Will

To start off, I am not a nutritionist and won't pretend to be. I did minor in nutritional sciences in college and have learned much through trial and error, but that is about it. Make sure to always get a doctor's approval before making any dietary changes. I have also read many books on the subject. Some were life changing and some I wouldn't suffer through again to save my own life! The underlying theme of this book is simplicity and effectiveness. This chapter is no different. I am a big believer in the bottom-line. Make sure it works and make sure people can understand how to apply it with zero confusion. There are so many "theories" on this subject it is nauseating. All of them have "testimonies" and people who believe in their special way so much it is almost like a religion. Some eating habits are highly complex and require weighing and measuring every single gram of macronutrients of every single meal. While others are much more broad in their approach. Again, we want simple and results! My favorite approach is foolproof. I call it the mirror technique. Skip out on the pricey body comp stuff and go into your bathroom strip down to your skimpies and look into the mirror. Unless you have been diagnosed with a serious mental disorder, like body dysmorphia, this actually works quite well. If you have excess body fat you will see it. If you look like a scrawny shaved bird you will easily be able to tell that you need to gain muscle. This is simple stuff folks! If you need to drop fat, you have two options. If you have lots of fat to lose, simply eat a little less each day and do the *Bradbury Muscle Course*. Aim to reduce your daily calories by 300-500 per day (that's only about 3 slices of bread and 1 soda). This will help you lose roughly 1 pound per week through this diet strategy alone. Not to mention you've added the *Bradbury Muscle Course* workouts into your regimen of daily activity. Our program builds muscle like crazy and everyone with a brain knows that it takes calories to keep your muscles alive and well. Muscles burn up calories throughout the day. The healthiest and best way to boost your metabolism is by building lean muscle. If you have just a little fat to lose say less than 10 pounds, you can make the dietary adjustment if you want to. However, just doing the *Bradbury Muscle Course* will burn additional calories and build lean muscle mass, which also burns up calories. I'd recommend complete the 12-week program and then reassess if you need to drop calories or not before the next 12-week cycle. You will be amazed at how your body transforms. You and everybody else will notice a significant difference in your appearance.

If you are skinny the same rule applies except the exact opposite. Try to increase your daily calories by 300-500 per day and let the program work its magic. In dire cases, you may need to add in even more calories. A sure-fire way to do this is to drink a high-quality protein supplement with all of your meals. It should go without saying, but don't fall for the marketing hype and buy cheap protein powder unless you want intense farts and a bloated look. If you like to live dangerously, whatever you do, do not buy cheap protein powder and cheap toilet paper at the same time. You will immediately regret that decision. Anyways back on track, your muscles will love the abundant flow of high quality amino acids accompanying your meals and they will reward you by busting out of your shirt sleeves to show their appreciation. If you do this religiously your muscles will grow, grow and keep growing.

If you are one of those guys or gals who need a precise formula and numbers to be able to sleep at night, rest assured. You can lose roughly 1 pound of fat per week at will by simply cutting out 3,500 calories per week. That comes out to 500 calories per day (500cal x 7 days = 3,500cal). "Only 1 pound per week! My class reunion is in one month!" Easy there cowboy. Rome wasn't built in a day either. Your body is a little more complicated than a bowl of instant grits. There are 24 weeks in 6 months. What if I told you that you could lose 24 pounds of pure fat in just 6 months? Shooting for 1 pound per week will lead to a positive experience and transformation by maximizing lean muscle mass and sizzling off any extra fat. This is the logical approach that will give you lasting results. This is not a quick fix "yo yo" diet that will actually make you fatter over the long haul. Here is precisely how to do it. It's estimated in a pound of fat there is 3,500 calories. Theoretically, if you cut back on just 500 calories per day for 7 days you would reach the 3,500 calorie mark and erase 1 pound of fat. If you really want to geek out search "BMR calculator" on the internet. Use this tool to figure out your basal metabolic rate (BMR). Then make sure to account for your activity level by applying your BMR result to the Harris Benedict Equation. This will accurately give you an estimate of your daily caloric needs to maintain your current bodyweight. This is important to know exactly how many calories you actually need. There are many online calculators that are simple to use to figure this out. Majority of people grossly over or under estimate how many calories they actually need to reach their goal. Now, you just add or subtract 300-500 calories per day depending on your goal. It is a great idea to count all calories for a few weeks with a calorie counting book or app to make darn sure you are precisely hitting your numbers. This will give you a good idea of exactly how much food is X amount of calories.

Example:

- Male, 6-foot, 200 pounds, 20 years old
- Works out with weights intensely 4 days per week
- BMR is 2090.4
- Harris Benedict Equation (activity level): BMR X 1.55 (look online for all possible activity levels)
- Total daily calories needed to maintain weight, including activity factor: **3,240.12**

In this example, if he wanted to get leaner and drop excess body fat at roughly one pound per week, he would take his 3,240.12 daily caloric need and subtract 500. That will be his target until he reaches his desired leanness. His target to lean out would now become 2,740.12 calories per day.

If you want to lose 1 pound per week, decrease intake by 500 calories per day (500 calories x 7 days = 3500 calories).

If you want to lose 1 pound per 14 days, decrease intake by 250 calories per day (250 calories x 14 days = 3500 calories).

29

Exposed: The Big Snare of Extreme Low Calorie Diets

It is commonplace in our society of instant gratification to want something yesterday! Although this is always a fool's game. This approach never works. If it does it is just a temporary fix. The "more is better" attitude plagues the masses into severe frustration and leads to mass confusion. The erroneous thought is "if it says cutting 500 calories works for 1 pound of fat loss per week, what if I cut 1,000 calories per day? I must lose more faster!" Sorry, but you are wrong, dead wrong. If that approach actually worked then you could starve yourself for a few days and be good to go. Prepare yourself, this is the truth and what REALLY happens in extreme caloric deficiencies. Sometimes the truth can be haunting and in this case it is no different. Your body is an extremely smart creature and will do anything at all costs to preserve life and protect itself. As a result, when you start your extreme caloric deficiency diet your body quickly senses famine and starvation. It begins to quickly slough off any excess lean muscle it deems unnecessary at an alarming rate. This is because muscles use up calories to maintain size, but the body is sensing it needs the calories more than the muscles do for survival. So it gets rid of the muscle tissue to save calories for itself to survive this perceived famine. Even worse news, your fat storage enzyme concentrations begin to skyrocket! Higher levels of fat storage enzymes can't be good. Your body is gearing up to store anything it can get a hold of as fat because it is sensing long-term famine and starvation. Congratulations, your "miracle diet" just turned your body into an extremely efficient fat storing machine and destroyed all of your hard-earned muscle. A double whammy! This ugly cycle creates the dreaded "yo yo" effect we all see people go through with their bodyweight struggles. The poor soul starves themselves and loses lots of "scale" weight initially. Unfortunately, most of this scale weight loss is lean muscle tissue. Muscle is denser and weighs much more than fat. They may have lost 30 pounds like magic! However, to their dismay they are caught in the snare. Their fat storing enzymes are at their highest concentration ever. So when they inevitably resume a normal diet, even a healthy one, at some point their body is going to store literally everything it can as fat. This is an survival adaptation to protect itself from the next famine it may face. This causes astronomical fat gain. Over time the pour soul becomes fatter than ever! This book is not a weight loss book. However, at least you now know the dark truth of the common snare that leads people to the doom of severe obesity. Now let's get back to building muscle.

30

How to Eat for Maximum Muscle and Minimal Fat

Now that you know how simple it really is to lose or gain weight with a smart approach. Let's go over what to eat and when to eat it to maximize muscle growth. I repeat, I am not a registered dietitian and it is out of the scope of this book to provide detailed meal plans. I am going to give you general guidelines and accepted information to teach you how to maximize your food intake to build slabs of muscle and flense off any extra body fat. This is presented as an example of proven guidelines and not a diet prescription.

It must be understood the grave importance of protein and its major role in extreme muscle development. The body is in a constant state of creating new cells to replace the dying cells and protein plays a key role in this process. You must consume plenty of protein at proper intervals every single day without fail. If your body needs energy and amino acids and you are not providing it through food, it will cannibalize your hard earned muscle to get it! The last thing you need is for your own body to eat up all of your muscle. Frequent, high protein meals are optimal. Aim for 4-6 meals per day as this is superior to just 3 meals per day. If you are looking to gain weight simply add a protein shake to every meal. If you learn just one thing from this book let it be this: NEVER, EVER SKIP BREAKFAST! This is a rookie mistake that leads to muscle loss, poor performance and fat gain.

As you can imagine, the process of digestion and absorption of food is a delicate and synchronized process. Your body has a lengthy process to properly breakdown and digest food. It precisely choreographs digestive enzymes and bodily functions to complete digestion from mouth to elimination. It is imperative to always allow at least 2-3 hours between meals to let your body fully digest and absorb your food optimally. Another common mistake millions make is eating a good solid meal and then come back 30 minutes later to "snack" on something silly. This foolish act totally disrupts the vital digestion sequence of the original meal. All of the nutrients from the original meal you thought you would benefit from now will not be digested correctly and will be wasted. Sit down, eat your meal and then don't eat anything for 2-3 hours. If you are currently an avid "snacker" now, you will be amazed at your improved energy and recovery once you begin to allow your body to actually absorb the food you are eating. I'm not going to give you a dissertation on what to eat. There are a few extreme strength and physique athletes that have had great success with what would be considered "bad" diets. For the mass majority of people, however, it is my strong belief that if you put in the right fuel that you will earn a stellar result. The opposite also holds true that if you put garbage in, you'll get garbage out. For 99.9% of the population the guidelines below will put you on the fast track to a superb physique.

BRADBURY MUSCLE COURSE DIETARY GUIDELINES

- Meet daily protein needs by eating lean animal proteins (meat, eggs, milk) and a high-quality protein supplement. One gram of protein per pound of bodyweight is optimal for muscle building.
- Each meal should contain: Lean Protein, Natural Starchy Carbohydrate, Natural Fibrous Carb, and a small amount of healthy fat. Example meal: Chicken Breast, Rice, Salad with Olive Oil for dressing.
- Muscles are mostly made of water. Drink lots of plain water to maximize performance, muscle pumps and recovery. Urine should always be a very light yellow color.
- Carbohydrates are the body's preferred fuel choice. Supply them in ample amounts to fuel your hardcore training sessions. Eat an adequate amount to fuel training, but not too much to store body fat. After 6PM, eat fibrous carbs only or no carbs at all to keep body fat low and to improve sleep quality.
- Fats pack the largest caloric punch per gram. This can be useful for someone needing to gain weight. Stick to fats from avocados, nuts, olive oil and especially fish oil. Remember, meats, eggs and milk contain fat so there is no reason to go overboard looking for ways to increase fat intake.
- Eat a large raw salad at least once daily. This can boost protein synthesis!
- Fiber is your friend. Make sure to get roughly 25-35 grams per day through fiber-rich food and/or fiber supplementation.
- Eat 4-6 high protein meals per day. Allow at least 2-3 hours in between to maximize nutrient absorption and optimal digestion.
- Calories are the gas pedal or brakes to gaining weight. If you want to get bigger you must eat more. If you want to shed excess fat you must eat less. Generally, 300-500 calories more/less per day works great to gain or lose weight in an appropriate manner. Remember, more is not necessarily better.
- Minimize, if not completely eliminate, highly processed and sugary foods. If you absolutely cannot live without these types of food, make sure to consume them within one hour after your workout to re-fill glycogen stores. Remember, discipline works so drop the junk to enhance your results.

It is important to learn how to balance daily nutrition:

- 1 gram of protein contains 4 calories
- 1 gram of carbohydrate contains 4 calories
- 1 gram of fat contains 9 calories
- 1 gram of alcohol contains 7 calories

Most people seeking a muscular transformation thrive on a daily intake that consists of:

50% of Calories from Carbohydrates
30% of Calories from Protein
20% of Calories from Fats

Calculate your BMR and add in activity level. Then take the total calories needed per day and make adjustment (up or down 300-500) for your goal. Then figure out how much from each macronutrient you need by multiplying total calories by the percentage of each macronutrient.

Example: BMR including activity level is 2600 calories.

2600 X .5 = 1300 calories from carbohydrate needed per day

1300 / 4 = 325 grams of carbohydrates needed per day

I hate to break it to you, but developing the perfect nutrition program is crafted through trial and error. It would be foolish and irresponsible to write out a detailed eating plan in this book. Many people have certain food allergies that can be mild or severe in nature. Also, everybody lives a different lifestyle. Some work an inactive desk job, while others lift heavy metal all day in a foundry. Armed with the mirror technique and the ability to calculate your BMR you will have a beacon through the dark night. Combined with the guidelines provided you will certainly find your way. The most important ingredient is an unwavering discipline. You must stay the course. Do not succumb to frequent temporary temptations that will lead you astray. If you can stay the path your body will reward you with results you once thought unimaginable.

31

The Cheat Meal Sham

A few years back "Cheat Meals" became fashionable. I for one gave it a whirl for awhile. The idea is that you eat healthy and "clean" for many days and then splurge yourself into oblivion on your designated cheat meal. At the cheat meal, you can eat whatever you want and as much as you want. The idea was wonderful. Something to look forward to and getting to eat all those delicious treats was a great time. This was to supposedly "shock" your body and boost your metabolism which made some sense. At first, I loved eating "clean" for several days and then acting like a selfish five year old on their birthday eating a bunch of junk food. Being a bottom-line guy, I tracked my progress and analyzed the results. I began to notice that my cravings for more junk food increased intensely making it harder to stick to my scheduled "clean" eating days. That might have been the powerful influence of sugar and foods artificially designed to taste delicious. I also noticed a severe slump in energy during the week and I can only think that it may have been caused from the stress of my body trying to process all that junk. I even noticed a lousy mood and a negative state of mind. Last but certainly not least, I started noticing an increase in body fat. That reality of increasing body fat was the end of the "cheat meal" era for me. It obviously did not work and provided no real benefits. Now, you shouldn't be the weirdo not eating with family and friends at holidays. Go ahead and have some fast food, desserts and such sparingly and always in moderation. If you are serious about achieving a superior physique, you cannot afford the drawbacks of a full-blown cheat meal. It makes zero sense to take 2 steps forward and 3 steps back. Enjoy those foods in moderation and you will be fine. Instead of 10 cookies shoot for one or two. Partaking in a cheat meal is a setback to the results you've been working so hard to get. Go out to eat, enjoy something sensible in moderation and enjoy the experience. People who earn an outstanding physique do so through hard work, consistency and discipline. Above all you must have discipline and I believe that the idea of a splurging cheat meal is an undisciplined act. It is an undisciplined action that can lead to an undisciplined snowball effect. Don't fall victim to the sham that is the cheat meal. Always enjoy tasty foods occasionally in moderation. Never let one gluttonous meal lay savage your potential results.

32

The Supplement Puzzle

The supplement industry, just like any industry, has it's fair share of con men. To make more profit they cheapen production costs and deliver you a lesser quality product to put into your body. To make even steeper profit margins some companies fill their bottles and jugs with sorry ingredients you wouldn't even want to feed to your dog. Hiding behind a fancy label and highly compensated endorsers many people fall victim to all the hype. The only result they receive is just another empty promise and a slimmer wallet. Supplements are big money! In any business, the more money it seems like you can make the more hucksters come out of the woodwork to try to tap into the profits. They will slash prices by filling their bottles with junk in a effort to fool the consumer. Cheaper is never better. Haven't you noticed that you always get exactly what you pay for? There have probably been a dozen new supplement companies started in the short time it took you to read this paragraph. So how does a person wisely maneuver through all of this mess and find a high-quality supplement? What should you look for to avoid making an expensive mistake? Luckily, this endeavor is not too terribly difficult. You must look for a company that has integrity. Most of the time sorry companies don't stand the ultimate test, the test of time. They may fool you once, but if their product sucks customers will not come back. Sooner or later they disappear. Bad companies are usually a flash in the pan and flee just as quickly as they came onto the scene. Search to find a company that has been around a good while. A company that is over twenty years old means they have stood the test of time. Do your own research and find a proven winner. You must do your due diligence as the bioavailability of your supplement is vital. What exactly is bioavailability? Bioavailability is just a fancy word that shows how much of your supplement actually gets absorbed and utilized by your body and how much of it is wasted. If it is made of junky ingredients your body cannot digest and absorb it. High-quality products or nothing should be your motto. You could buy a huge jug of protein and think you are supplementing 60 grams per day. However, you bought the cheap stuff and may be only absorbing 15 grams or less! Therefore the suggested list below must be of the highest quality or you are wasting your money and not reaping the benefits.

SUPPLEMENT SHOPPING LIST

- Creatine Product
- Protein Powder
- Amino Acid Product
- Carbohydrate + Protein Powder

- Pre-Workout Product
- Maca Root Product
- Multivitamin
- Omega 3 Fish Oil

These products will help you enhance your results and perform optimally day in and day out. You don't need supplements to get results, however, the right supplements are proven to amplify results and optimize your health. This list will lead to much faster recovery, enhanced performance, and more muscle! Feel free to add or subtract supplements on an as needed basis. These are the proven basics and they will work.

SUPPLEMENT TIMELINE ***CONSULT A DOCTOR AND ALWAYS USE AS DIRECTED BY MANUFACTURER***

1. Multivitamin and Fish Oils with breakfast
2. Protein Powder with meals and as needed to meet protein needs
3. Amino Acid Product between meals
4. Pre-Workout before workout (no-brainer!)
5. Creatine Product with Carbohydrate + Protein Powder with post workout meal
6. Maca Root Product use as directed by manufacturer
7. Fish Oils with dinner

33

The Elephant in the Room: Anabolic Steroids

In all honesty, this is a tough topic to tackle. I could have taken the easy route, stuck my head in the sand, and easily left this portion out. However, many people wonder about this subject. They see people and think "I wonder if he is juicing?" or they don't know where to find legit help and get themselves in a very dangerous situation. **Let's get one thing straight from the get-go, I do not recommend the use of anabolic steroids.** Personally, I have never used illegal steroids. I have witnessed a great deal of people acquire an incredibly muscular physique completely drug free. I have also seen people amass incredible feats of strength without steroids. To me the potential risks of undesirable side effects and legal concerns always outweighed the possible rewards. This is simply my opinion and I have no hard feelings towards people who choose to use anabolic steroids. The potential nasty side effects and extraordinary expense of these agents have never appealed to me. Did you know that some people spend upwards of 2 to 4 thousand dollars per month on these drugs? That adds up to a whopping 24K to 48K per year! To some it is well worth the cost if it is vital to their competitive career and their quest for titles in bodybuilding or powerlifting. As of late, there is a vast array of hormone boosting treatments available. Like anything, some people believe wholeheartedly in these new treatments and others think it is a complete sham and doesn't work at all. Although steroid use is an individual choice, I propose a different route. How about you keep the 24K per year in your pocket. Then utilize a sound training program that is proven to deliver maximal muscle gains coupled with a disciplined nutrition approach and see what happens. Stack that with high-quality supplementation and you will be well on your way. You will achieve a physique only dreamed of by the guy using illegal drugs, stacked like tortillas, with a sorry training program and junky nutrition. I believe, without a shadow of a doubt, that with diligent hard work and equipped with the *Bradbury Muscle Course* you can achieve a steroid-like physique. You'll also be healthier in the long haul versus mingling with potentially dangerous pills and/or shots. You will be able to enjoy a natural muscular body for years and years to come. Your body won't grow and then quickly wither from cycling off steroids. You will build a body that will look awesome all of the time. Now for most of us we don't ever have a desire to cross that line. We believe in a natural approach to building as much muscle as possible. However, there are others who are willing to cross that line. They are willing to invest lots of money and potential health threats for the vision of an extreme physique. It would be a disservice to disregard these individuals because they are reading this book too searching for training help. It would be foolish and dishonest to say that steroids do not work. If you look at the top bodybuilders today versus the ones of yesteryear the changes are undeniable. With the advancement in "steroid science" and the meticulous "stacking" of these powerful compounds bodybuilders look superhuman nowadays. It seems bigger is best as it is now commonplace to see 300+ pound guys with extremely low body fat levels. Back in the golden age, the majority were between 180-240 pounds at contest time. So as far as muscle size goes, proper drug use (if there is such a thing) does work. Imagine adding in a powerful program that actually works with or without drugs! If you do choose to use drugs, perform the *Bradbury Muscle Course* for superior results. The miraculous size and strength gains seen on natural lifters will undoubtably be enhanced by the anabolic effects of these extreme compounds. I care about you. It truly hurts my heart hearing of a life-halting illness or the tragedy of an early death due to drug abuse. Sadly, this is all too common with steroid use. In the quest of extreme muscle enhancement there are those who succumb to reckless "stacking" and abusing these potent substances. This commonly ends in a tragedy. Another fellow iron warrior down for the count. TRAGEDY! The saddest thing is that most of the time it could have been avoided. From the bottom of my heart please promise me one thing. Can you do this one thing for you, your family, and your friends? If you choose to go the unnatural route only do so under a doctor's close supervision. Frequent blood testing can prevent you from becoming the next tragedy. Close monitoring is the safest way. Please be vigilant and as long as you use these agents do us all a favor and periodically get checked out by a doctor. Check your ego at the door and get this done at all costs, it could very well save your life one day. Now, thank you for going through this difficult subject. Please take to heart what is written here. It could very well save lives. In conclusion, I always recommend going the natural route without using potentially dangerous compounds. I believe a smart program, disciplined nutrition and good ole fashioned elbow grease is all the ingredients you need to become a muscle building machine.

34

Watch Your Back

It is all too common to see people become overzealous about their new workout program and become reckless with their training. They push themselves way too hard at the beginning just to find themselves quitting a short time later. In recent years, the introduction of "for time" workouts and a do or die attitude has amplified this problem. Most of the time the PR's people do achieve with this approach are simply "newbie" gains and cease within one year or so of training. This stalling out is due to their workouts not specializing on continuing to improve on that specific task. While this type of intensity and motivation can be helpful, it must be carefully used in moderation. Like anything, going totally overboard everyday is a recipe for disaster. There is a big difference from training hard and being just plain reckless. Reckless people don't last very long and are always injured in some way. Who wants to live injured all the time? It's no secret that the very best physiques took years to develop. The very best physiques are reserved for the people who always train smart and can do so long term. If you find yourself getting hurt often, even with minor injuries, within the first 3 years you are way off the mark. If you develop your body sensibly and with a smart program, like the *Bradbury Muscle Course*, you should experience incredible improvements with little to no problems. However, if you "thrash" yourself day in and day out you will have lots of problems and become an orthopedic Doctor's dream. The most common injuries seen around the industry are the low back, hips, shoulders and knees. Most of the time, this is due to repetitive overuse injuries and/or muscular weaknesses causing imbalances. Have you ever experienced a back spasm? If you have you surely understand why keeping your low back strong and healthy is an absolute must. Nothing is more crippling than a powerful back spasm. The good news is by spending time developing every muscle in a focused and balanced manner you can prevent many of these pitfalls. The *Bradbury Muscle Course* targets every fiber of every muscle with compound and isolation movements to bring them up to their maximum potential. Bigger, stronger muscles means more stability around joints and the ability to withstand more punishment than scrawny, weak muscles. Have you ever wondered why you never see a skinny and frail running back in professional football? It is because the skinny and frail running backs either adapt by getting bigger and stronger to withstand the punishment or they get left behind in the pee wee or high school ranks. Your body is the same way. Unless you live in bubble wrap and sit in a locked room all day, you will at some point experience some degree of punishment. You may trip and fall while playing basketball. You may be water skiing and take a nasty spill. You may have to lift a heavy flower pot that your wife wants "over there." You may be playing with your kids and have to cut sharply to avoid getting tagged. Ask any physical therapist and they will tell you that people get hurt in the oddest ways. Sadly, many people can't experience the simple exhilarations of life because they sorely lack physical fitness. This is why you must develop your muscles! You don't want to retire one day just to realize you can't do anything because you have become weaker and weaker over the years at your day job. Building your muscles bigger and stronger one by one will give you the freedom and confidence to live life to it's fullest everyday. You will get injured less often and if you do it will heal up fast. You will notice that you will not get sick as often. Imagine, all these potential benefits and many more because you chose to build muscle. I could write another entire book just on the countless success stories and testimonies regarding this topic of the freedoms of living a fitness lifestyle. Now it is my strong belief that you should never injure yourself in a workout because of careless actions. Pushing yourself to reach new levels of muscular development is commonplace in our program. However, by implementing sensible increases, periodization techniques, and built in recovery phases, the *Bradbury Muscle Course* sets you up to perform at the highest intensity in the safest manner possible. The *Bradbury Muscle Course* is a very safe program designed for longevity. You will achieve quick and long

term gains. Every exercise builds on the others to work with a high level of synergy. Synergy means that all parts are working together congruently to deliver a desirable outcome. By systematically putting synergy in your corner you will experience greater improvements with much less risk. Let me say one more time, it makes zero sense to hurt yourself because of ignorance during a workout. This program is about building you up and not about landing you in a surgeon's office. As aforementioned, your lower back and hips are a very important part of your body. Ask anyone who has suffered years of back pain and they will surely shed some doom and gloom about their experience. This program is designed to build your

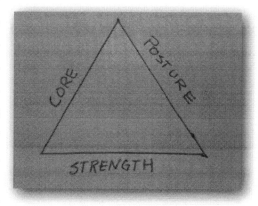

back muscles to be strong. A strong back is a healthy back. Proper posture is also a major player to overall back and spine health. You will notice your posture will vastly improve performing this program. You will stand taller and sit with better posture. Last but not least, core strength plays a key role in keeping your low back healthy. Everyone needs to have very strong abs. These three elements: <u>STRENGTH</u>, <u>POSTURE</u>, <u>CORE</u> make up what I call the Triad of Back Health. This is also an idea of utilizing the true power of synergy. If any part of the triad is underdeveloped, overall back health will undoubtably suffer at some level. Remember, a chain is only as strong as it's weakest link. You only get one spine and it's a good idea to take care of it. The *Bradbury Muscle Course* capitalizes on the idea of the triad in it's unique programming. You will notice lots of focused back work to boost strength. You will notice substantial posture improvements. Lastly, our "core focus" portion of the workouts use only the best of the best of proven core exercises. We shy away and eliminate movements that cause grinding or twisting of your spine to bits. The core focus sections will improve all parts of the triad. In error, many people blindly follow the latest "ab trend" on social media and not only do they not get any results, but they unknowingly cause unrepairable damage to their spine! Don't succumb to this idiocy. Endless twisting and sit-up movements is like putting a meat grinder to your delicate spinal structures. Our program employs only the smartest core movements that will strengthen and more importantly balance your entire core for enhanced performance. You will develop a rock hard midsection designed for peak performance. The *Bradbury Muscle Course* is all about results and longevity. If you are anything like me, you want to lift heavy iron forever. This program is uniquely designed to allow you to keep improving for many years to come. Real physical fitness is not a flash in the pan quick fix, rather it is a lifelong commitment to being able to live an exceptionally vibrant life due to your success in maintaining a superb level of physical fitness.

35

King of Core: Turkish Get Up

The Turkish Get Up (TGU) is so important that it deserves to be displayed in it's very own chapter. As you will see this is a major player in our "core focus" portions of the *Bradbury Muscle Course*. Not only am I going to teach how to perform it correctly with ease. We will also go over why it is such a vital piece to our muscle building puzzle. The TGU is one of the best exercises you can do for your body, especially while you are packing on lots of muscle. When your body adds lean muscle mass it must adapt to it's new size and shape by re-developing full-body coordination. Imagine doing a pullup as a skinny dude weighing 145 versus a pullup weighing 225 with less than 8% body fat. The additional 80 pounds of lean muscle mass will surely make the pullup happen. However, now being much bigger you still need to move an additional 80 pounds!

Also, all of the levers are slightly different since you've added lots of muscle mass to your frame. In a sense, your body must then re-learn the pattern of the movement. This is one reason why I absolutely love the TGU. When you start adding muscle to your frame you will need to work on flexibility, stability and full body coordination. The TGU is excellent at maximizing all three in one single exercise. It takes coordination to even perform one rep without any additional weight. It takes excellent coordination and full body spatial awareness (proprioception) to perform a rep with a weight held above your head. The TGU is your go to exercise to build a bulletproof core. It works about every muscle in your body, but really challenges your abs and obliques. It will help your shoulders move through a full range of motion and maintain stability throughout the entire movement. The TGU gets an A+ for maintaining peak shoulder health. Your core will also learn how to brace, stabilize a load, and do so under dynamic circumstances. Therefore, it is a forgone conclusion that to maintain full body awareness and coordination while adding lots of lean muscle the TGU is your golden ticket. This movement will keep you agile, flexible and coordinated. It will also bombproof your shoulders to keep them healthy for the onslaught of heavy pulls and presses of the *Bradbury Muscle Course*.

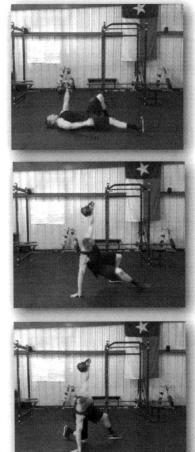

Now let's go over how to do a TGU correctly. Unfortunately, many people do them heinously wrong. This is a very complex movement with a lot of moving parts. Please understand, the TGU must be mastered before adding any weight.

Do not attempt to add weight too soon. Stick with sensible progressions just like any other movement. Also, do not rush this movement. Hit each point with precision and under full control. Never bend your arm! You cannot hit yourself in the head with your hand with a straight arm and the same rule applies when holding a kettlebell or dumbbell. If you get out of control, move the kettlebell or dumbbell as far away from your body as possible and drop it to the ground. Do not try to save it and keep it in a position to where it could fall on any part of your body. When you switch the kettlebell or dumbbell to the other side do so by bringing it down real close to your chest and switch it to your other hand. Do not attempt to switch hands up high above your head, throat and chest area as this is a serious accident waiting to happen.

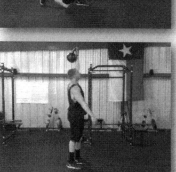

How to perform a TGU:

Start by laying down with a kettlebell or dumbbell in one hand
Stare at the KB/DB the entire movement
On the same side as the KB/DB, bend that leg up to a 90 degree angle (just remember same side as KB/DB bend that leg)
Push the KB/DB up until arm is straight and keep it straight the entire movement
Drive the elbow on the opposite side down into the ground
Raise up until you transition your base of support from the elbow to your palm
Now raise your hips as high as possible
Swing your leg all the way back and through into a proper lunge position
Perform a lunge and make sure to keep arm straight
Stand up tall
Now to finish rep one go back down the exact way you came up
Lunge back, go down to your palm and swing leg back
Go down under control to elbow and then finally back to laying down into start position.

A couple of tips to maximize your TGU. Make sure to brace your core the entire movement. Never allow yourself to lose tightness in your midsection during any portion of the TGU. Always look directly at the kettlebell or dumbbell the entire movement. The act of staring at the KB/DB helps to maintain balance and maximizes spatial awareness. Plus, it's a good idea to keep an eye on the weight over your head. Never allow your ego to get in the way and try to do too much weight before you are prepared for it. You can get a wonderful core workout by doing just bodyweight TGU's. This exercise works literally every muscle in your body and provides quite the conditioning experience due to the oxygen debt you surely will encounter. Truly, it is a burpee on steroids. Make sure to be precise and under control the entire time. Never rush a TGU. The TGU is a staple in our "core focus" portions of the *Bradbury Muscle Course*. The "core focus" portion is key to promoting low back health, a rock hard midsection and keeping your full body in balance to enhance performance. Remember, you are only as strong as your weakest link. Many programs grossly neglect focused core work and can lead to less than optimal performance and many times a crippling low back injury. By adding in core focused programming and the TGU into your arsenal you are sure to see bigger lifts, a chiseled midsection and a healthier low back.

36

Cardio Question

"What about cardio?" is a common question I get. Most of the stigma still lingers from the 70's and 80's and the aerobics craze. Cardio is a buzzword nowadays and some people think you must have a dose of it before or after lifting weights to have a truly effective and balanced workout. I strongly differ in opinion. I am the leanest and most muscular I've ever been and I do 4 weight training sessions per week following the *Bradbury Muscle Course* precisely. In addition, I have my diet dialed in for my goal at all times. I have achieved these results despite a bizarre sleep schedule. This is due to getting up at 3AM Monday through Friday and working early mornings and evenings as a fitness professional. To make matters worse, fitness bracelets that track steps and such have become more fashionable. Nowadays, people are even more in tune with cardio than ever. They feel like if they don't walk at least 10,000 steps per day their whole life is in shambles and they are on the road to obesity. This mindset is utterly false and you should be counting reps, not steps. Don't get me wrong for some people aerobics is a great solution. However, you are in it to win it and you know now that resistance training is vital for a transformation. In fact, you are reading the best book ever written on how to grow muscle. If you are a big believer in cardio, listen with an open mind and hear me out on this. At the highest levels of society, aerobics has been ingrained into our minds to think it is the only way to get healthy by many influences. Masses of people are heavily confused by this idea. Let's use common sense for once on this subject. First off, what exactly is aerobics? Aerobics 101 sounds like the first class you'd take in flight school. Aerobics, by definition, is any activity that takes place with the use of oxygen. Anaerobic activity (e.g. 1 rep max) takes place without oxygen. Believe it or not, you are performing aerobics by sitting quietly reading this book (no jogging suit required). You perform aerobics while sleeping and walking to get the mail. Virtually any living human is performing aerobics all day. So if someone asks, "do you do any aerobics?" You say, "Why yes I do! Everyday!" It's a no-brainer that you can only survive a short time without oxygen. The idea that aerobics "burns" fat is also questionable. There are even certain training intensities called "fat-burning" zones. While it is true that performing aerobics burns calories and can burn off body fat, there is a much bigger problem lingering for you. Aerobics is also extremely proficient at burning off lean muscle too. Too much of a good thing and you'll be sloughing off hard earned muscle by the pound. A quick web search of "endurance athletes" and you'd be hard pressed to find an 18+" bicep. Since your mission is to build muscle you'd be best to leave extra aerobic work alone. Actually, avoid it like the plague.

"Won't I get fat if I don't do extra cardio and just lift weights?" The truth is that the only biological way to gain fat is to consume too many calories. It is completely moronic to think that lifting weights builds fat. If you eat more calories than you burn off over time, you will start to gain fat. Here is the key to your quandary: MUSCLE BURNS

CALORIES. The healthiest and best way to boost your metabolism is by building lean muscle. The more muscle you acquire the more calories your body will burn off throughout the day. Common sense tells us that if you burn more calories per day by adding more muscle you will not get fat and in fact become leaner and leaner over time. This is what I refer to as "The Tipping Point." The tipping point idea takes affect when you build so much muscle your body essentially turns into a caloric furnace every single day. This leveraged approach to burning calories is because of your vast increase in lean muscle mass. Your body is burning loads of calories everyday automatically thanks to your muscles. It like the old saying "the rich just get richer!" The exact same idea applies. You add more muscle and fat begins to disappear almost effortlessly. People will start to wonder if you have some secret diet pill or magic juice and they will start pulling straws. When the answer has been staring them in the face the whole time! Focus on building as much lean muscle mass as possible and allow the tipping point to run it's course. You will find yourself becoming leaner and leaner month after month, year after year. Getting leaner and adding more muscle month after month. Imagine that! Talk about a win-win. Again, it only makes common sense if you focus all of your energy on growing muscle that your body will flense away fat if your diet remains the same. Just make sure you are dialed in and eating enough to support your daily needs and not too much that it will store as fat.

If you perform the *Bradbury Muscle Course* correctly and precisely adhere to the prescribed rest periods you will develop a conditioning level that most could only dream of. Take note of how out of breath you become on your 1st leg day! However, if you need extra conditioning work due to a lousy diet or wanting to get as lean as possible (see how to get ripped in 6 weeks chapter), avoid long, slow cardio at all costs. Instead, opt to do intervals executed at a very high intensity where the work portion is maximum output followed by an easy rest period. It is proven, high intensity intervals are superior for building your conditioning level, burning fat and minimizing muscle loss versus long, slow cardio. If you play sports, feel free to supplement the *Bradbury Muscle Course* with sport-specific conditioning 2-3 times per week (see FAQ's). If you are looking to build as much muscle as possible, skip all forms of cardio and follow the *Bradbury Muscle Course* precisely and control body fat levels with your diet. Believe it or not, the saying that "abs are built in the kitchen" is absolutely true!

37

How to Get Ripped in 6 Weeks

There will come a time when you will want to get absolutely shredded. Deep cuts, striations, and veins pop-ping everywhere will show off your newly earned muscle mass like no other. You will drop body fat levels to competition levels and achieve razor sharp definition. It is important to understand that you need to make sure to build a substantial amount of muscle with the *Bradbury Muscle Course* before doing this 6-week cycle for extreme leanness. I would recommend doing 3 to 4 full 12-week cycles of the *Bradbury Muscle Course* before embarking on this endeavor. A scrawny guy with low body fat doesn't have the same impact as an extremely muscular guy with low body fat levels. It is important to understand that performing the *Bradbury Muscle Course* and following a proper eating regimen will give you a very lean and muscular build alone. This 6-week phase is utilized to achieve extremely low body fat levels and should only be done only once or twice a year. The masses will undoubtably embark on this expedition 6 weeks before spring break, class reunions and the like. I cannot stress enough that you should be lean year-around and never allow your diet to increase your fat levels. Do not be foolish and attempt to "bulk" up adding noticeably more and more fat along the way. You can eat more to gain muscle, but avoid eating too much and gaining fat. All that fat you gain from over-eating, you will at some point have to diet long term to get rid of it the right way. You should walk around everyday with a very muscu-lar and lean physique. If you follow this program correctly, you'll never have to worry again about a shirts and skins pickup game, rather you will welcome them. You can add in this 6-week program as a supplement to the *Bradbury Muscle Course* to enhance your definition to jaw dropping levels.

How this works is really simple. You will work to **adjust your diet** to support and maintain lean muscle mass and drop body fat percentage even lower. You will **add in high intensity conditioning** protocols 1-3 times per week in addition to the *Bradbury Muscle Course*. You will also **ramp up your high-quality amino acids** supple-ment intake to help preserve lean muscle mass. Tanning is optional, however, tan skin shows off muscularity bet-ter than pasty skin.

First things first, how to eat during this 6-week lean out phase. You must continue to eat ample amounts of lean protein to minimize muscle loss. Strive to maintain the 1 gram per pound of bodyweight recommendation and maybe a touch more during this very intense phase. Keep protein intake from lean, high-quality meats, eggs and high-quality protein supplements only. Light canned tuna in water can be very helpful during this time as a fast, high protein food. You will also aim to drop 200-400 calories from your current total daily intake. Try to mainly drop those calories from carbohydrates and fats. In summary, your protein intake stays the same or increases and your carbohydrate and fat intake drops. Most of the caloric deficit should come from carbohydrates. Here is a crucial key, only eat natural starchy carbohydrates before and immediately (within 1 hour) after your workout. Any other time you can eat fibrous carbs such as salad, broccoli or vegetables with other meals if you so choose. You will need carbs for energy before your workout and then immediately after to restore your glycogen levels. Executing this nutrient timing precisely will give you energy to power through intense workouts and enhance recovery. I would also strongly suggest using a fiber supplement everyday during this 6 weeks to enhance digestion. Every one lives with a different schedule. This next suggestion is for the masses who work all day and go to bed around 9-10pm. You must avoid starchy carbohydrates at all costs after 6pm. This will help drop body fat levels and give you a natural growth hormone spike while sleeping to support protein synthesis and recovery. Remember, growth hormone is famously known to help you get lean! During this phase, you must also drink tons of water. Do not be shy here. Water is extremely anabolic and helps boost protein synthesis. You really can't get too much water. Protein synthesis at a time of caloric deficiency is your golden ticket.

It has been proven time and time again that long, slow cardio activities (jogging, running long distances, swimming endless laps, etc) are not your friend if you are trying to maximize lean muscle mass. Some people do these activities for overall health and wellness. Others really enjoy these activities and I am not trying to discredit their endeavors. However, if you want muscle and lots of it you need to avoid these activities like the bubonic plague. Taking a nice 20-30 minute leisurely walk is okay to get the blood flowing, get some fresh air and enhance recovery. Other than a refreshing walk, take my advice and pass on the long, slow stuff. It has been proven in the trenches and in the fancy labs that high intensity interval training is superior for burning fat while preserving muscle. HIIT is the optimal conditioning method to flense off extra body fat while sparing lean muscle tissue. This is the only type of conditioning you will do during this phase. It is imperative to work at a maximal output during the work portion of the interval. Then you will go at an easy pace during the rest portion of the interval. The age old saying, that you get out what you put in rings true here. Your results depend solely on how hard you are willing to push yourself. I prefer activities that are very simple in nature for interval work. It is never wise to do highly complex movements while experiencing extreme fatigue because technique will suffer. An airbike, rowing machine or sprinting is hard to beat. You can really redline yourself and you won't have to slow down to analyze technique or risk an injury. My very favorite interval comes from Dr. Izumi Tabata and his Tabata Protocol. This 4 minute gut-busting interval is simple and flat out works. It comprises of 20 seconds of max effort work followed by 10 seconds of rest (easy pedaling, rowing, or walking/jogging). You then repeat this for a total of 8 intervals. If you push yourself, this interval will put you on the fast track to shedding off fat. You will also experience an euphoria like non other as you can imagine. Another interval I love to utilize is purely for your burst and power system. It is also a beast if you really give it all you've got on the work portion. The second interval option is what I call the Power Interval. You perform 10 seconds of max effort work followed by 20 seconds of very low intensity activity. You will also do this for 8 intervals. The key on this one is you really got to make the 10 seconds count! You gotta make it an absolutely gut-busting 10 seconds. You can really ramp up the power output on this one. When should you do your intervals? If possible, do the interval work of your choosing first thing in the morning before eating breakfast. Then wait 3 or more hours to do your assigned *Bradbury Muscle Course* workout for the day. This is optimal and the best option! Or you can do your interval work on your rest day first thing in the morning. If this isn't an option you can do the *Bradbury Muscle Course* workout and then wait 3 or more hours and then return to do your interval. This lean out phase only lasts 6 weeks so make necessary adjustments to make it happen! If none of that works with your schedule, you can perform your interval before or after your *Bradbury Muscle Course* workout for the day. Ladies do the interval work prior to hitting the weights. Men do the interval work after hitting the weights. This last option isn't ideal, however, since you will undoubtably be able to work at a much higher intensity if you have a 3+ hour break in between the workout and interval work.

INTERVALS TO KEEP MUSCLE AND LOSE FAT:

Tabata Interval Protocol - 20W/10R X 8 intervals

Power Interval Protocol - 10W/20R X 8 intervals

W is work; R is rest; 10 or 20 is in seconds

There is no reason to make it any more complex than that. Pick one protocol or mix them up for 1-3 days per week during the 6 weeks. This will put your body into an oxygen debt like no other and burn even more calories throughout the day. All of this works together and will remove any extra body fat. At the same time, utilizing these protocols you will preserve your lean muscle mass as much as possible. Big muscles, minimal fat is always a win-win! A note on recovery, please do not go overboard during this 6 week lean out phase. If you are an advanced trainee and train with big poundages you may only need to do 1 interval per week to get desired effects. If you are a beginner you can probably get away with 2-3 intervals per week. Remember, more is not necessarily better! One thing about these high intensity intervals is that they do cause stress that the body must recover from. If you do them too frequently and are hitting the weights hard you could severely over-stress your body. If you over-stress your body and your CNS, your performance will go down the tubes and you will start to lose muscle mass at an alarming rate. Remember, you are cutting calories as well so be careful to not over do it by doing too many days of intervals. I'd recommend the first time through this 6 week cutting phase, just do 1 day of intervals per week for the 6 weeks and then reassess. If your diet is where it needs to be, that might be all it takes to get absolutely ripped. You can always add another day or two the next time you tackle this 6 weeks again.

Last but not least, make the amino your amigo. Be sure to ramp up your amino acid supplement intake during this 6 week phase. This will help you keep more of your hard earned muscle. It goes without saying, but you must use amino acids of the highest quality. Don't ever cut corners when it comes to quality versus cheap. Another great muscle sparing supplement is creatine. You should be already using this anyways, but if you haven't been now would be a good time to start. I get asked "is creatine a steroid?" all too often. No! This is another false myth that confuses people. Creatine is a completely natural ergogenic aid. It's so natural in fact, you can get creatine from eating a steak. I haven't seen a t-bone show up on any banned substance lists lately. Your body produces some creatine naturally. However, when dosed properly using a high quality creatine supplement you can enhance your performance and muscle mass considerably. Creatine is one of the most researched supplements out there and has high marks for the muscle builder. Make sure to drink plenty of water when using creatine to maintain hydration levels. In summary, ramp up those amino acids to preserve your muscle mass during this intense 6-week lean out period. Use a creatine product too for more insurance to protect from muscle loss. Wise supplementation will help you reach your goals faster and enhance your performance.

One final word, don't get it confused this 6-week lean out phase is not a miracle quick fix. If you have more than 10-15 pounds of fat to lose this is not for you… yet! I would recommend that you do the *Bradbury Muscle Course* and get your diet dialed in to get your fat levels down the right way first. You must build lots of lean muscle first before performing this portion to get desired effect. I always recommend working to achieve a lean, muscular physique year-round. Avoid junky "bulks" at all costs. If you want to build muscle eat more, but not so much that you notice fat increasing too. Noticeable fat increases are simply from consuming too much food. The only biological way to gain adipose tissue (ugly fat) is to eat too much food. This 6-week period is for someone who has already built a substantial amount of muscle with our program and has worked hard to have a low body fat percentage. Then to take it to the extreme and get lean as humanly possible they will perform this 6-week phase in addition to their *Bradbury Muscle Course* training. This will get them to competition-level definition. As mentioned earlier, I'd say do this hardening phase once or twice per year. For the rest of the year, tackle the *Bradbury Muscle Course* cycle after cycle to continue packing on lean mass and strength gains. Important Note: please understand when you are working at a calorie deficiency and adding in high intensity intervals that you may notice your strength levels dip. Do not be alarmed as this is completely normal. When you are performing this cutting phase your lifts on your strength focus will decrease in weight to some degree. That is okay as they will quickly return to normal levels and usually higher once you return to your normal regimen after this 6-week phase has concluded. For this 6-week phase your mission is to get as lean as possible. What you have in your hands is a proven way to get extremely ripped. Stick to the plan and use discipline and this will work wonders for you.

<u>WARNING</u>

Consult a doctor before embarking on the following training program. The *Bradbury Muscle Course* is a high intensity program that could possibly result in severe injuries or even death. The reader assumes any and all risks and responsibility for any and all damages resulting from this material. Please adhere to the program guidelines and recommendations closely. Make sure to have an attentive spotter and proper spotting mechanisms for all movements.

All rights reserved. The following program is intellectual property intended for only the reader who purchased this book. No part of this program can be reproduced or transmitted in any form or by any means, including social media, without written permission from the author.

Part 3: The Training Program

38

Bradbury Muscle Course

You will notice that in the *Bradbury Muscle Course* you will encounter three distinct phases. I believe it is important to go over each phase in detail so you understand what is going on. This will arm you with motivation to tackle each phase fiercely and watch those muscles start to grow. It is nothing short of incredible the changes you will see on your own body if you just work hard and stay committed.

PHASE 1:

Phase 1 is a 3 week wave of extremely high volume. This will utterly put your muscles into shock and they will respond by growing and growing a lot! The main exercise will be 5 sets of 10 reps. Utilizing 5 sets of 10 reps allows you ample practice time with each movement to really hone in your skills and develop critical lifting technique mastery. Accompanied with many other movements that will target literally every single fiber of every muscle. During this phase, many experience soreness in areas they did not even know existed. Imagine, how much more muscle you will grow when you train in this manner. A bit of warning, if you are brand new and just starting out you want to ease into this program. If you over do it at first, I can assure you crippling soreness. It is wise to take the first week light and easy to feel things out. Even if you take it super easy you will still get sore. Remember, more is not better and you must progress sensibly for maximal gains. Many will notice that they simply do not have the conditioning and stamina to complete the entire workout at first. This is okay and normal. Many have never worked at an output that will actually get them results. If your past workouts were 20 minutes or less, you'll be in for quite a shock. Don't worry, it will take no time at all until your body has acquired the superb conditioning required to complete the workouts. Always give it your best shot. If you feel like you've gave it your absolute all and still have exercises to do it's okay to pass on them for that day. Mark my words, you will complete all the exercises and sets next time around. Be sure to follow rest periods precisely. This will ensure an extreme hormonal response that will lead to even more muscle and fat burning. You will start to see noticeable differences in your physique in the first 3 weeks. If you are eating sensibly you will also see the fat literally melt off of your body as your muscles will begin to enlarge.

PHASE 2:

Enter the famous pyramid sets of 12,10,8,6,4 reps. Pyramids have been building incredible physiques for ages. Personally, this is my favorite phase although all phases must be included to make this one really shine. Now that your conditioning and technique is up to par thanks to the grueling phase 1, we can now get to the good stuff.

We can now focus on building insane amounts of lean muscle mass. Pyramids allow the body to work naturally into heavier and heavier weights every set. They provide plenty of volume and serve to bridge the gap between our high volume training to our lower volume, higher intensity training. All forms are required in moderation to train optimally for muscle growth. This phase will once again shock your muscles into more explosive growth. Your body will welcome the lower volume and heavier weights and reward you with more muscle. Your motivation will skyrocket when you see the heavy weights on the bar for the 6 and 4 rep sets. Performing a pyramid protocol is really quite simple. Perform 12 hard reps, then add a little weight and do 10 hard reps. Then you'll add some more weight and do 8 and so on until you do your heaviest set of 4 reps. Make sure to follow prescribed rest periods precisely. You will enjoy this phase because the visible results are now becoming undeniable. People will start to notice and ask questions. Stick to the plan of following the program precisely, eating for your goal and keep those results coming.

PHASE 3:

You've made it to the third and final phase, the heaviest phase of all. You will get to perform 5 sets of 5 reps on the main exercise. On the "Pump Focus" section intensity will be at an all time high. When you watch a fireworks show they always climax with a grand finale and this is no different. To take advantage of both types of muscle hypertrophy (myofibrillar and sarcoplasmic) you must hoist some heavy iron! Many programs out there forget this and make this error. You my friend are prepared and ready to tackle this phase. The fives will once again shock your muscles into further growth. Strength gains will also be evident as you have gotten much stronger throughout the program. The Repeated Effort Method will also get lots of playing time during this phase to drive even more adaptations and grow even more muscle. During week 11, you will get the opportunity to establish 1 to 5 rep maxes for the major lifts: Squat, Bench Press, Deadlift & Military Press. You get to choose if you want to do a 5 rep max or a 1 rep max or anywhere in between. If you don't really care about doing a 1 rep max, I'd suggest sticking with the 5 or 3 rep max. However, if you really want to know what your 1 rep max is, perform a 1 rep max. Any way you choose to go, this will be vital information to track your overall strength progress cycle to cycle.

A NOTE ON GROWTH WEEKS 4, 8, & 12:

Trust me, when you start out you will be very enthusiastic and will be strongly tempted to over do it on the Growth Weeks. Do not be foolish and do this. Have some discipline and drop the pre-workout supplements for this week and take it easy and follow the program exactly as it is written. Properly executed Growth Weeks are a vital part of our program and must be adhered to closely. If you do not follow Growth Weeks precisely your results will suffer. These weeks will allow you to practice movements with lighter loads and work on the mind to muscle connection. Most importantly, they will allow your body to fully recover. Not only your muscles, but your tendons, ligaments and nervous system will be allowed to fully recover and heal up completely. Your body will get a chance to supercompensate and grow bigger, stronger muscles, which is what you want isn't it? All of this works together with perfect timing. When the Growth Week ends you'll be biting at the bit to get back to the gym and hit the weights with an extreme intensity.

OPTIMAL TRAINING DAYS

Monday: Day 1

Tuesday: Day 2

Wednesday: REST

Thursday: Day 3

Friday: Day 4

Saturday: REST

Sunday: REST

There are many different options. Make it fit your schedule. This arrangement above is optimal to maximize results and recovery.

All workouts have a specific identity code to help you to identify your current location. This is proven to make things simple when looking back in your journals and logging weights. Write the code for each workout clearly in your journal for quick reference. It also tells you exactly where you are in the program in an instant.

W = week

D = day

GW = growth week

Example: Week 5, Day 2 workout would be scripted W5D2

IMPORTANT NOTICE

Each workout contains 3 parts:

1. Strength Focus
2. Pump Focus
3. Core Focus

Make sure to complete all 3 parts of every workout. In the following pages, the *Bradbury Muscle Course* is written out in great detail to make things simple for you. Make sure you always check the next page to make sure you can see the entire workout.

W1D1

STRENGTH FOCUS (2-3 minutes rest between sets)

Bench Press 5x10

Incline Dumbbell Press 4x10

Weighted Dips 3x10

PUMP FOCUS (45 seconds rest between sets)

Flat Dumbbell Chest Fly 3x11

Flat Dumbbell Chest Fly 1x20

Barbell Cheat Curls 12,10,8,6

Zottman Curls 3x11

Concentration Curls 3x11

Overhead Dumbbell French Press 4x11

Triceps Cable Pushdown Straight Bar 1x30

CORE FOCUS (15-30 seconds rest between sets)

Plank Hold 2 x 60 seconds

Side Plank Hold 2 x 30 seconds per side

W1D2

STRENGTH FOCUS (2-3 minutes rest between sets)

Back Squat 5x10

Dumbbell Lunges 4x10 per leg

PUMP FOCUS (45 seconds rest between sets)

Belt Squat or Leg Press 3x11

Goblet Squat 1x20

Glute Ham Raise or Leg Curl 4x11

Sissy Squats 3x20

Perform Calf Blast Twice

CORE FOCUS (15-30 seconds rest between sets)

McGill Curl-Up 10 reps (5/leg; Hold each rep 10 seconds)

Hanging Leg Raises 3x15

Reverse Hyper or Back Extensions 3x15

W1D3 REST

W1D4

<u>STRENGTH FOCUS</u> (2-3 minutes rest between sets)

Narrow Grip Bench Press 5x10

Dumbbell Shoulder Press 4x10

<u>PUMP FOCUS</u> (45 seconds rest between sets)

Lying Triceps Extensions 4x11

Dumbbell Kickbacks 3x11

Triceps Rope Cable Pushdown 1x30

Dumbbell Front Raise 3x11

Dumbbell Lateral Raise 3x11

Dumbbell Bent Over Lateral Raise 3x11

Y-T-I Shoulder Complex 1x8/position

<u>CORE FOCUS</u> (15-30 seconds rest between sets)

Ab Wheel Rollout 3x10

Bodyweight Turkish Get Up 3x8 (4 per side)

W1D5

<u>STRENGTH FOCUS</u> (2-3 minutes rest between sets)

Deadlift 3x5

Power Shrug 3x5

Romanian Deadlift 3x10

<u>PUMP FOCUS</u>

Dumbbell Shrugs 3x11

T-Bar Row 4x11

Dumbbell Row 1 x max reps

Chin-ups 3x11

Wide Lat Pulldowns 2x11

Straight Arm Dumbbell Pullovers 2x15

Incline Bench Curls 3x11

Preacher Curls 3x11

Preacher Curls 1x20

Perform Calf Blast Once

No core focus today.

W1D6 REST

W1D7 REST

This concludes week 1 of the *Bradbury Muscle Course.*

W2D1
STRENGTH FOCUS (2-3 minutes rest between sets)
Incline Bench Press 5x10
Dumbbell Bench Press 4x10
Bodyweight Dips 3 x max reps

PUMP FOCUS (45 seconds rest between sets)
Slight Incline Fly 3x11
Slight Incline Fly 1x20
Barbell Cheat Curls 12,10,8,6
Zottman Curls 3x11
Hammer Curls 1 x max reps
Overhead Dumbbell French Press 4x11
Straight Bar Cable Triceps Pushdown 2x20

CORE FOCUS (15-30 seconds rest between sets)
Plank Hold 2 x 60seconds
Side Plank Hold 2 x 30seconds

W2D2
STRENGTH FOCUS (2-3 minutes rest between sets)
Front Squat 5x10
Bulgarian Split Squats 4x10 per leg

PUMP FOCUS (45 seconds rest between sets)
Belt Squat or Leg Press 3x11
Belt Squat or Leg Press 1x30
Glute Ham Raise or Leg Curl 4x11
Romanian Deadlift 3x8
Perform Calf Blast Twice

CORE FOCUS (15-30 seconds rest between sets)
McGill Curl-Up 10 reps (5/leg; Hold each rep 10 seconds)
Hanging Leg Raises 3x15

W2D3 REST

W2D4
STRENGTH FOCUS (2-3 minutes rest between sets)
Narrow Grip Bench Press 5x10
D.E. Push Press 5x3 (60 seconds rest) ***see dynamic effort method section***
Standing Military Press 3x10

PUMP FOCUS (45 seconds rest between sets)
Lying Triceps Extensions 4x11
Dumbbell Kickbacks 3x11
Dumbbell Kickbacks 1 x max reps
Barbell Front Raise 3x11
Dumbbell Lateral Raise 3x11
Dumbbell Bent Over Lateral Raise 3x11
Barbell Upright Row 2x20

CORE FOCUS (15-30 seconds rest between sets)
Ab Wheel Rollouts 5x10
Turkish Get Ups 3x2 (1 per side)

W2D5
STRENGTH FOCUS (1-2 minutes rest between sets)
Power Shrug 5x3
Farmer's Walk 3x100ft

PUMP FOCUS (45 seconds rest between sets)
Dumbbell Shrugs 2 x max reps
Bent-Over Barbell Row 4x11
Dumbbell Row 1 x max reps
Wide Pullups 4 x max reps
Wide Lat Pulldown 1x30
Back Extensions 2x15
Incline Dumbbell Curls 4x11

Preacher Curls 3x11

Concentration Curls 15,12,10 per arm

No core focus today.

W2D6 REST

W2D7 REST

This concludes week 2 of the *Bradbury Muscle Course.*

W3D1

STRENGTH FOCUS (2-3 minutes rest between sets)

Bench Press 5x10

Incline Dumbbell Press 4x10

Weighted Dips 3x10

PUMP FOCUS (45 seconds rest between sets)

Flat Dumbbell Chest Fly 3x11

Flat Dumbbell Chest Fly 1x20

Barbell Cheat Curls 12,10,8,6

Zottman Curls 3x11

Concentration Curls 3x11

Overhead Dumbbell French Press 4x11

Triceps Cable Pushdown Straight Bar 1x30

CORE FOCUS (15-30 seconds rest between sets)

Plank Hold 2 x 60seconds

Side Plank Hold 2 x 30seconds per side

W3D2

STRENGTH FOCUS (2-3 minutes rest between sets)

Back Squat 5x10

Dumbbell Lunges 4x10 per leg

PUMP FOCUS (45 seconds rest between sets)

Belt Squat or Leg Press 3x11

Goblet Squat 1x20

Glute Ham Raise or Leg Curl 4x11

Sissy Squats 3x20

Perform Calf Blast Twice

CORE FOCUS (15-30 seconds rest between sets)

McGill Curl-Up 10 reps (5/leg; Hold each rep 10 seconds)

Hanging Leg Raises 3x15

Reverse Hyper or Back Extensions 3x15

W3D3 REST

W3D4

STRENGTH FOCUS (2-3 minutes rest between sets)

Narrow Grip Bench Press 5x10

Dumbbell Shoulder Press 4x10

PUMP FOCUS (45 seconds rest between sets)

Lying Triceps Extensions 4x11

Dumbbell Kickbacks 3x11

Triceps Rope Cable Pushdown 1x30

Dumbbell Front Raise 3x11

Dumbbell Lateral Raise 3x11

Dumbbell Bent Over Lateral Raise 3x11

Y-T-I Shoulder Complex 1x8/position

CORE FOCUS (15-30 seconds rest between sets)

Ab Wheel Rollout 3x10

Turkish Get Ups 3x4 (2 per side)

W3D5

STRENGTH FOCUS (2-3 minutes rest between sets)

Deadlift 3x5

Power Shrug 3x5

Romanian Deadlift 3x10

PUMP FOCUS

Dumbbell Shrugs 3x11

T-Bar Row 4x11

Dumbbell Row 1 x max reps

Chin-ups 3x11

Wide Lat Pulldowns 2x11

Straight Arm Dumbbell Pullovers 2x15

Incline Bench Curls 3x11

Preacher Curls 3x11

Preacher Curls 1x20

Perform Calf Blast Once

No core focus today.

W3D6 REST

W3D7 REST

This concludes week 3 of the *Bradbury Muscle Course.*

GROWTH WEEK

Note: Growth Weeks are specially designed to allow your body to fully restore and recover. This week will lead to greater muscle growth and muscle density. For maximum effectiveness, follow protocol exactly. It is a great idea to cease use of pre-workout supplements this week. Your pump will not be as intense as usual due to the decrease in volume and intensity. DO NOT overexert yourself or do extra exercises during Growth Weeks.

W4D1-GW

STRENGTH FOCUS (2-3 minutes rest between sets)

Incline Bench Press 3x10 @ 70% Week 2's Weight

Dumbbell Bench Press 3x10 @ 70% Week 2's Weight

Bodyweight Dips 2 x max reps @ 70% Week 2's Reps

PUMP FOCUS (45 seconds rest between sets)

Slight Incline Fly 3x11 @ 80% Week 2's Weight

Barbell Curls 10,8 @ 80% Week 2's Weight

Zottman Curls 2x11 @ 80% Week 2's Weight

Overhead Dumbbell French Press 3x11 @ 80% Week 2's Weight

Straight Bar Cable Triceps Pushdown 1x20 @ 80% Week 2's Weight

CORE FOCUS (15-30 seconds rest between sets)
Plank Hold 1 x 60seconds
Side Plank Hold 1 x 30seconds

W4D2-GW
STRENGTH FOCUS (2-3 minutes rest between sets)
Front Squat 3x10 @ 70% Week 2's Weight
Bulgarian Split Squats 2x10 per leg @ 70% Week 2's Weight

PUMP FOCUS (45 seconds rest between sets)
Belt Squat or Leg Press 2x11 @ 80% Week 2's Weight
Glute Ham Raise or Leg Curl 2x11 @ 80% Week 2's Weight
Romanian Deadlift 2x8 @ 70% Week 2's Weight
Calf Raises 3x20 @ 80% Week 2's Weight

CORE FOCUS (15-30 seconds rest between sets)
McGill Curl-Up 6 reps (3/leg; Hold each rep 10 seconds)
Hanging Leg Raises 2x15
Reverse Hyper or Back Extensions 2x20 light

W4D3-GW REST

W4D4-GW
STRENGTH FOCUS (2-3 minutes rest between sets)
Narrow Grip Bench Press 3x10 @ 70% Week 2's Weight
D.E. Push Press 3x3 (60 seconds rest) @ Same as Week 2's Weight
Standing Military Press 2x10 @ 70% Week 2's Weight

PUMP FOCUS (45 seconds rest between sets)
Lying Triceps Extensions 3x11 @ 80% Week 2's Weight
Dumbbell Kickbacks 2x11 @ 80% Week 2's Weight
Barbell Front Raise 2x11 @ 80% Week 2's Weight
Dumbbell Lateral Raise 2x11 @ 80% Week 2's Weight
Dumbbell Bent Over Lateral Raise 2x11 @ 80% Week 2's Weight

CORE FOCUS (15-30 seconds rest between sets)
Ab Wheel Rollouts 3x10
Bodyweight Turkish Get Ups 2x6 (3 per side)

W4D5-GW

<u>STRENGTH FOCUS</u> (1-2 minutes rest between sets)

Power Shrug 3x3 @ 70% Week 2's Weight

Farmer's Walk 2x100ft @ 70% Week 2's Weight

<u>PUMP FOCUS</u> (45 seconds rest between sets)

Dumbbell Shrugs 1x15 light

Bent-Over Barbell Row 3x11 @ 80% Week 2's Weight

Wide Pullups 3 x max reps

Back Extensions 1x15 @ 80% Week 2's Weight

Incline Dumbbell Curls 3x11 @ 80% Week 2's Weight

Preacher Curls 2x11 @ 80% Week 2's Weight

Concentration Curls 15,12 per arm @ 80% Week 2's Weight

No core focus today.

W4D6-GW REST

W4D7-GW REST

This concludes week 4 GROWTH WEEK of the *Bradbury Muscle Course*.

W5D1

<u>STRENGTH FOCUS</u> (2-3 minutes rest between sets)

Bench Press 12,10,8,6,4

Incline Dumbbell Press 12,10,8,6

Weighted Dips 10,8,6

Bodyweight Dips 1 x max reps

<u>PUMP FOCUS</u> (45 seconds rest between sets)

Flat Dumbbell Chest Fly 15,12,10,8,20

Barbell Cheat Curls 12,10,8,6

Zottman Curls 3x11

Concentration Curls 15,12,10 per arm

EZ Bar French Press 3x11

Straight Bar Triceps Cable Pushdown 2x20

Straight Bar Triceps Cable Pushdown 1 x max reps

CORE FOCUS (15-30 seconds rest between sets)
Plank Hold 2 x 60seconds
Side Plank Hold 2 x 30seconds per side

W5D2
STRENGTH FOCUS (2-3 minutes rest between sets)
Back Squat 12,10,8,6,4
Barbell Walking Lunges 12,10,8,6 per leg

PUMP FOCUS (45 seconds rest between sets)
Belt Squat or Leg Press 3x11
Belt Squat or Leg Press 20,30
Glute Ham Raise or Leg Curl 4x11
Sissy Squats 3x25
Perform Calf Blast Twice

CORE FOCUS (15-30 seconds rest between sets)
McGill Curl-Up 10 reps (5/leg; Hold each rep 10 seconds)
Hanging Leg Raise 3x15
Reverse Hypers or Back Extensions 3x15

W5D3 REST

W5D4
STRENGTH FOCUS (2-3 minutes rest between sets)
Narrow Grip Bench Press 12,10,8,6,4
Dumbbell Shoulder Press 12,10,8,6

PUMP FOCUS (45 seconds rest between sets)
Lying Tricep Extensions 15,12,10,8
Incline Single Arm Dumbbell French Press 3x11 per arm
Triceps Cable Rope Pushdown 20,30
Dumbbell Bent Over Lateral Raise 3x11
Dumbbell Front Raise 3x11
Dumbbell Lateral Raise 12,15
Dumbbell Lateral Raise 1 x max reps immediately followed by a max time hold with dumbbell held 2 feet from body

CORE FOCUS (15-30 seconds rest between sets)
Turkish Get Up 4x4 (2 per side)
Ab Wheel 3x10

W5D5
STRENGTH FOCUS (2-3 minutes rest between sets)
Deadlift 5,4,3,2
Power Shrug 5,4,3
Weighted Pullups 10,8,6

PUMP FOCUS (45 seconds rest between sets)
Double D Handle Lat Pulldown 3x11
T-Bar Row 15,12,10,8
Dumbbell Row 1 x max reps
Barbell Shrugs 3x11
Incline Dumbbell Curls 15,12,10,8
Preacher Curls 3x11
Reverse Curl Cluster: 5 reps followed by 10-15 seconds rest repeat for 5 minutes
Perform Calf Blast Once

No core focus today.

W5D6 REST

W5D7 REST

This concludes week 5 of the *Bradbury Muscle Course.*

W6D1
STRENGTH FOCUS (2-3 minutes rest between sets)
Incline Bench Press 12,10,8,6,4
Dumbbell Bench Press 12,10,8,6
Bodyweight Dips 3 x max reps

PUMP FOCUS (45 seconds between sets)
Slight Incline Fly 15,12,10,8,20
Dumbbell Alternating Curl 4x11 per arm
Hammer Curls 15,12,10,8

Bench Dips with Plate(s) in lap 15,12,10

Bench Dips with Plate(s) in lap 1 x max reps

Straight Bar Cable Pushdown Cluster: 6 reps followed by 10-15 seconds rest repeat for 5 minutes

CORE FOCUS (15-30 seconds rest between sets)

Plank Hold 2 x 60 seconds

Side Plank Hold 2 x 30 seconds

W6D2

STRENGTH FOCUS (2-3 minutes rest between sets)

Front Squat 12,10,8,6,4

Bulgarian Split Squat 12,10,8,6 per leg

PUMP FOCUS (45 seconds rest between sets)

Sissy Squats 50,40,30,20,10

Glute Ham Raise or Leg Curls 5x11

Perform Calf Blast Twice

CORE FOCUS (10-15 seconds rest between sets)

Hanging Ab Raise 5x15

McGill Curl-Up 10 reps (5/leg; Hold each rep 10 seconds)

W6D3 REST

W6D4

STRENGTH FOCUS (2-3 minutes rest between sets)

Narrow Grip Bench Press 12,10,8,6,4

D.E. Push Press 5x3 (45 seconds rest)

Standing Military Press 12,10,8,6

PUMP FOCUS (45 seconds rest between sets)

EZ Bar French Press 15,12,10,8

Dumbbell Kickbacks 20,15,12

Dumbbell Kickbacks 1 x max reps

Giant set (no rest between exercises):

Barbell Front Raise, 11 reps

Barbell Upright Row, 15 reps (same weight as front raise)

Bent Over Lateral Raise, 11 reps

Rest 45 Seconds

Complete Giant Set 5 times

CORE FOCUS (30 seconds rest)

Turkish Get Ups 3x4 (2 per side)

Ab Wheel Rollouts 4x10

W6D5

STRENGTH FOCUS (2-3 minutes rest between sets)

Farmer's Walk 4x100 feet

Power Shrug 5,4,3,2

Dumbbell Shrug Cluster: 7 reps followed by 10-15 seconds rest repeat for 5 minutes

PUMP FOCUS (45 seconds rest in between sets)

Bent Over Row 15,12,10,8

Dumbbell Row 1 x max reps

Wide Grip Pullups complete 50 reps in as few sets as possible

Double D Handle Lat Pulldown 15,12,10,30

Run the Rack Dumbbell Curls -

perform 6 curls with heaviest dumbbells possible,

immediately grab next lighter dumbbells and perform max reps,

immediately grab next lighter dumbbells and perform max reps,

continue this pattern until you have gone through whole rack

Concentration Curls 15,12,10,10

Single Leg Calf Raises 3x20

No core focus today.

W6D6 REST

W6D7 REST

This concludes week 6 of the *Bradbury Muscle Course.*

W7D1

STRENGTH FOCUS (2-3 minutes rest between sets)

Bench Press 12,10,8,6,4

Incline Dumbbell Press 12,10,8,6

Weighted Dips 10,8,6

Bodyweight Dips 1 x max reps

PUMP FOCUS (45 seconds rest between sets)
Flat Dumbbell Chest Fly 15,12,10,8,20
Barbell Cheat Curls 12,10,8,6
Zottman Curls 3x11
Concentration Curls 3x15 per arm
EZ Bar French Press 15,12,10,8
Straight Bar Triceps Cable Pushdown 2x20
Straight Bar Triceps Cable Pushdown 2 x max reps

CORE FOCUS (15-30 seconds rest between sets)
Plank Hold 2x60 seconds
Side Plank Hold 2x30 seconds per side

W7D2
STRENGTH FOCUS (2-3 minutes rest between sets)
Back Squat 12,10,8,6,4
Barbell Walking Lunges 12,10,8,6 per leg

PUMP FOCUS (45 seconds rest between sets)
Belt Squat or Leg Press 3x11
Belt Squat or Leg Press 20,30
Glute Ham Raise or Leg Curl 4x11
Sissy Squats 4x15
Perform Calf Blast Twice

CORE FOCUS (15-30 seconds rest between sets)
Hanging Leg Raise 3x15
Reverse Hypers or Back Extensions 3x15
McGill Curl-Up 10 reps (5/leg; Hold each rep 10 seconds)

W7D3 REST

W7D4
STRENGTH FOCUS (2-3 minutes rest between sets)
Narrow Grip Bench Press 12,10,8,6,4
Dumbbell Shoulder Press 12,10,8,6

PUMP FOCUS (45 seconds rest between sets)

Lying Tricep Extensions 4x11

Incline Single Arm Dumbbell French Press 3x11 per arm

Triceps Cable Rope Pushdown 20,30

Dumbbell Bent Over Lateral Raise 3x11

Dumbbell Front Raise 3x11

Dumbbell Lateral Raise 12,15

Dumbbell Lateral Raise 1 x max reps immediately followed by a max time hold with dumbbell held 2 feet from body

CORE FOCUS (15-30 seconds rest between sets)

Turkish Get Up 6x2 (1 per side)

Ab Wheel 3x10

W7D5

STRENGTH FOCUS (2-3 minutes rest between sets)

Deadlift 5,4,3,2

Power Shrug 5,4,3

Weighted Pullups 10,8,6

PUMP FOCUS (45 seconds rest between sets)

Double D Handle Lat Pulldown 3x11

T-Bar Row 4x11

Dumbbell Row 1 x max reps

Barbell Shrugs 3x11

Incline Dumbbell Curls 15,12,10,8

Preacher Curls 3x11

Reverse Curl Cluster 5 reps followed by 10-15 seconds rest repeat for 5 minutes

Perform Calf Blast Once

No core focus today.

W7D6 REST

W7D7 REST

This concludes week 7 of the *Bradbury Muscle Course.*

GROWTH WEEK

Note: Growth Weeks are specially designed to allow your body to fully restore and recover. This week will lead to greater muscle growth and muscle density. For maximum effectiveness, follow protocol exactly. It is a great idea to cease use of pre-workout supplements this week. Your pump will not be as intense as usual due to the decrease in volume and intensity. <u>DO NOT overexert yourself or do extra exercises during Growth Weeks.</u>

W8D1-GW

<u>STRENGTH FOCUS</u> (2-3 minutes rest between sets)
Incline Bench Press 12,10,8 @ 70% of Week 6's Weight
Dumbbell Bench Press 12,10,8 @ 70% of Week 6's Weight
Bodyweight Dips 1 x max reps @ 70% of Week 6's Reps

<u>PUMP FOCUS</u> (45 seconds between sets)
Slight Incline Fly 15,12,10 @ 80% of Week 6's Weight
Dumbbell Alternating Curl 3x11 @ 80% of Week 6's Weight
Hammer Curls 12,10 @ 80% of Week 6's Weight
Bench Dips with Plate(s) in lap 15,12,10 @ 80% of Week 6's Weight
Straight Bar Triceps Pushdown 2x20 @ 80% of Week 6's Weight

<u>CORE FOCUS</u> (15-30 seconds rest between sets)
Plank Hold 1x60 seconds
Side Plank Hold 1x30 seconds

W8D2-GW

<u>STRENGTH FOCUS</u> (2-3 minutes rest between sets)
Front Squat 12,10,8 @ 70% of Week 6's Weight
Bulgarian Split Squat 12,10,8 @ 70% of Week 6's Weight

<u>PUMP FOCUS</u> (45 seconds rest between sets)
Sissy Squats 3x15
Glute Ham Raise or Leg Curl 3x11 @ 80% of Week 6's Weight
Calf Raises 3x20 @ 70% of Week 6's Weight

<u>CORE FOCUS</u> (10-15 seconds rest between sets)
Hanging Ab Raise 2x15
McGill Curl-Up 6 reps (3/leg; Hold each rep 10 seconds)

W8D3-GW REST

W8D4-GW

STRENGTH FOCUS (2-3 minutes rest between sets)

Narrow Grip Bench Press 12,10,8 @ 70% of Week 6's Weight

D.E. Push Press 3x3 (45 seconds rest) Same Weight As Week 6

Standing Military Press 12,10,8 @ 70% of Week 6's Weight

PUMP FOCUS (45 seconds rest between sets)

EZ Bar French Press 15,12,10 @ 80% of Week 6's Weight

Dumbbell Kickbacks 15,12 @ 80% of Week 6's Weight

Barbell Front Raise 2x11 @ 80% of Week 6's Weight

Barbell Upright Row 2x15 @ 80% of Week 6's Weight

Bent Over Lateral Raise 2x11 @ 80% of Week 6's Weight

CORE FOCUS (30 seconds rest)

Bodyweight Turkish Get Ups 20 total reps (10 per side)

Ab Wheel Rollouts 3x10

W8D5-GW

STRENGTH FOCUS (2-3 minutes rest between sets)

Farmer's Walk 2x100 feet @ 70% of Week 6's Weight

Power Shrug 5,4,3 @ 70% of Week 6's Weight

Dumbbell Shrug 20,15,12 @ 80% of Week 6's Weight

PUMP FOCUS (45 seconds rest in between sets)

Bent Over Row 12,10,8 @ 80% of Week 6's Weight

Wide Grip Pullups 3 x max reps

Double D Handle Lat Pulldown 15,12 @ 80% of Week 6's Weight

Dumbbell Curls 3x11 @ 80% of Week 6's Weight

Concentration Curls 12,10 @ 80% of Week 6's Weight

Reverse Hypers 2x11

Calf Raises 3x25

No core focus today.

W8D6-GW REST

W8D7-GW REST

This concludes week 8 GROWTH WEEK of the *Bradbury Muscle Course.*

W9D1

STRENGTH FOCUS (2-3 minutes rest between sets)

Bench Press 5x5

Incline Dumbbell Press 4 x max reps

Weighted Dips 3x5

PUMP FOCUS (45 seconds rest between sets)

Slight Incline Dumbbell Chest Fly 3x11 Immediately follow each set with Pushups for Max Reps

Concentration Curls 4x11

Zottman Curls 2x11

Barbell Cheat Curl Strip Set - Start with a weight you can do for 6 reps with max effort. Perform 6 reps and immediately strip 5-20lbs off and then perform max reps. Then immediately strip another 5-20lbs off and perform max reps again. Repeat this pattern until bar is completely empty.

Lying Triceps Extension 4x11

Bench Dips with Plate(s) in Lap 3x11

CORE FOCUS (15-30 seconds rest between sets)

Plank Hold 2x60 seconds

Side Plank Hold 2x30 seconds per side

W9D2

STRENGTH FOCUS (2-3 minutes rest between sets)

Back Squat 5x5

Dynamic Effort Back Squat 8x2 @ 60% 1RM (30 seconds rest between sets)

can be performed regular or to a box.

PUMP FOCUS (45 seconds rest between sets)

Glute Ham Raise or Leg Curl 5x11

Complete 5 Times: Belt Squat or Leg Press perform 15 reps immediately followed by Sissy Squats to failure

Perform Calf Blast Twice

CORE FOCUS (15-30 seconds rest between sets)

Hanging Leg Raise 3x15

Reverse Hypers or Back Extensions 3x15

McGill Curl-Up 10 reps (5/leg; Hold each rep 10 seconds)

W9D3 REST

W9D4

STRENGTH FOCUS (2-3 minutes rest between sets)

Narrow Grip Bench Press 5x5

Run The Rack Dumbbell Shoulder Press:

perform 6 Shoulder Presses with heaviest dumbbells possible,

immediately grab next lighter dumbbells and perform max reps,

immediately grab next lighter dumbbells and perform max reps,

continue this pattern until you have gone through the entire rack

PUMP FOCUS (45 seconds rest between sets)

Dumbbell Bent Over Lateral Raise 4x11

Dumbbell Lateral Raise 3x11

Barbell Front Raise Cluster perform 5 reps followed by 10-15 seconds rest repeat for 5 minutes

Dumbbell Lying Tricep Extensions 4x11

Incline Single Arm Dumbbell French Press 3x11 per arm

Incline Single Arm Dumbbell French Press 1 x max reps

CORE FOCUS (15-30 seconds rest between sets)

Turkish Get Ups 4x4 (2 per side)

Ab Wheel 3x10

W9D5

STRENGTH FOCUS (2-3 minutes rest between sets)

Deadlift 3x3

Power Shrug 3x3

Weighted Pullups 3x5

PUMP FOCUS (45 seconds rest between sets)

Giant set (no rest between exercises):

Pullups, max reps

T-Bar Row, 11 reps

Hammer Curls, 11 reps per arm

Rest 45 Seconds

Complete Giant Set 5 times

Dumbbell Row 2 x max reps

Incline Dumbbell Curls 3x11

Preacher Curl Cluster 5 reps followed by 10-15 seconds rest repeat for 5 minutes

Perform Calf Blast Once

No core focus today.

W9D6 REST

W9D7 REST

This concludes week 9 of the *Bradbury Muscle Course.*

W10D1

<u>STRENGTH FOCUS</u> (2-3 minutes rest between sets)

Incline Bench Press 5x5

Dumbbell Bench Press 4 x max reps

Bodyweight Dips 3 x max reps

<u>PUMP FOCUS</u> (45 seconds rest between sets)

Dumbbell Flat Chest Flys 5x11

<u>Giant set (no rest between exercises):</u>

EZ Bar French Press, 6 reps

Bench Dips with Plate(s) in lap, 12 reps

Dumbbell Kickbacks, 24 reps

Rest 45 Seconds

Complete Giant Set 5 times

Barbell Cheat Curls 3x8

Concentration Curls 4x11

Zottman Curls 2x15

<u>CORE FOCUS</u> (15-30 seconds rest in between sets)

Plank 2x60 seconds

Side Plank 2x30 seconds

W10D2

<u>STRENGTH FOCUS</u> (2-3 minutes rest between sets)

Front Squat 5x5

D.E. Front Squat 8x2 @ 60% 1RM (30 seconds rest between sets)

can be performed regular or to a box

PUMP FOCUS (45 seconds rest between sets)
Giant set (no rest between exercises):
Barbell or Dumbbell Walking Lunge, 6 reps per leg
Goblet Squats, 12 reps
Sissy Squats, 15 reps
Rest 45 Seconds
Complete Giant Set 5 times
Glute Ham Raise or Leg Curl 15,12,10,8
Perform Calf Blast Twice

CORE FOCUS (15-30 seconds rest between sets)
Hanging Leg Raise 100 reps in as few sets as possible

W10D3 REST

W10D4
STRENGTH FOCUS (2-3 minutes rest between sets)
Narrow Grip Bench Press 5x5
D.E. Push Press 6x3 (45 seconds rest between sets)
Military Press 3x5

PUMP FOCUS (45 seconds rest between sets)
Barbell Front Raise 15,12,10,8
Dumbbell Lateral Raise 3x11
Bent Over Lateral Raise 15,12,10,8
Lying Tricep Extensions 4x11
Straight Bar Tricep Cable Pushdowns 20,15,12,10
Straight Bar Tricep Cable Pushdowns 1 x max reps

CORE FOCUS (15-30 seconds rest between sets)
Turkish Get Ups 6x2 (1 per side)
Ab Wheel Rollouts 3x10

W10D5
STRENGTH FOCUS (2-3 minutes rest between sets)
Power Shrug 3x3
Farmer's Walk 3x100ft immediately followed by dumbbell shrugs for max reps

PUMP FOCUS (45 seconds rest)

Complete 50 Wide Grip Pullups in as few sets as possible

Double D Handle Lat Pulldown 15,20,30

Bent Over Barbell Row 4x11

Dumbbell Row 1 x max reps

Giant set (no rest between exercises):

Barbell Cheat Curls, 6 reps

Incline Dumbbell Curls, 12 reps

Preacher Curls, 24 reps

Rest 45 Seconds

Complete Giant Set 5 times

No core focus today.

W10D6 REST

W10D7 REST

This concludes week 10 of the *Bradbury Muscle Course.*

W11D1

STRENGTH FOCUS (2-3 minutes rest between sets)

Bench Press work up to establish a 1-5 rep max

Incline Dumbbell Press 4 x max reps

Weighted Dips 3x5

Bodyweight Dips 1 x max reps

PUMP FOCUS (45 seconds rest between sets)

Slight Incline Chest Fly 20,15,12,10,8

Barbell Cheat Curls 12,10,8,6

Zottman Curls 3x11

Concentration Curls 3x15

Straight Bar Triceps Cable Pushdown 20,15,12

Straight Bar Triceps Cable Pushdown 1 x max reps

Single Arm Incline French Press 4x11

CORE FOCUS (15-30 seconds rest between sets)
Plank 2x60 seconds
Side Plank 2x30 seconds

W11D2
STRENGTH FOCUS (2-3 minutes rest between sets)
Back Squat work up to establish a 1-5 rep max

PUMP FOCUS (45 seconds rest between sets)
Dumbbell Walking Lunges 15,12,10,8 reps per leg
Belt Squat or Leg Press 3x11
Belt Squat or Leg Press 1x20
Glute Ham Raise or Leg Curl 4x11 immediately follow each set with 20 Sissy Squats
Perform Calf Blast Twice

CORE FOCUS (15-30 seconds rest between sets)
Hanging Leg Raise 3x15
Reverse Hyper or Back Extensions 3x15

W11D3 REST

W11D4
STRENGTH FOCUS (2-3 minutes rest between sets)
Military Press work up to establish a 1-5 rep max
Narrow Grip Bench Press 5x5

PUMP FOCUS (45 seconds rest)
Dumbbell Shoulder Press 4x11
Bent Over Lateral Raise 3x11
Dumbbell Front Raise 3x11
Upright Barbell Row 3x11
Bench Dips with Plate(s) in lap 4x11
Dumbbell or EZ Bar Lying Tricep Extensions 15,12,10,8
Rope Triceps Cable Pushdowns 3x20

CORE FOCUS (15-30 seconds rest between sets)
Turkish Get Up perform 30 reps (15 per side) with moderate weight with minimal rest

W11D5

STRENGTH FOCUS (2-3 minutes rest between sets)

Deadlift work up to establish a 1-3 rep max

Weighted Pullup work up to establish a 5 rep max

PUMP FOCUS (45 seconds rest between sets)

Wide Grip Lat Pulldown 3x11

Wide Grip Lat Pulldown 1 x max reps

T-Bar Row 15,12,10,8

Dumbbell Shrugs 3 x max reps

Hammer Curls 15,12,10,8

Incline Dumbbell Curls 3x11

Preacher Curls 3x15

Perform Calf Blast Once

No core focus today.

W11D6 REST

W11D7 REST

This concludes week 11 of the *Bradbury Muscle Course.*

GROWTH WEEK

Note: Growth Weeks are specially designed to allow your body to fully restore and recover. This week will lead to greater muscle growth and muscle density. For maximum effectiveness, follow protocol exactly. It is a great idea to cease use of pre-workout supplements this week. Your pump will not be as intense as usual due to the decrease in volume and intensity. DO NOT overexert yourself or do extra exercises during Growth Weeks.

W12D1-GW

STRENGTH FOCUS (2-3 minutes rest between sets)

Incline Bench Press 3x5 @ 70% of Week 10's Weight

Dumbbell Bench Press 3 x max reps @ 70% of Week 10's Reps

Bodyweight Dips 2 x max reps @ 70% of Week 10's Reps

PUMP FOCUS (45 seconds rest between sets)

Dumbbell Flat Chest Flys 3x11 @ 80% of Week 10's Weight

EZ Bar French Press 3x11 @ 70% of Week 10's Weight

Bench Dips with Plate(s) in lap 2x12 @ 80% of Week 10's Weight

Dumbbell Kickbacks 2x15 @ 80% of Week 10's Weight

Barbell Cheat Curls 10,8 @ 80% of Week 10's Weight

Concentration Curls 2x11 @ 80% of Week 10's Weight

Zottman Curls 2x15 @ 80% of Week 10's Weight

CORE FOCUS (15-30 seconds rest in between sets)

Plank 1x60 seconds

Side Plank 1x30 seconds

W12D2-GW

STRENGTH FOCUS (2-3 minutes rest between sets)

Front Squat 3x5 @ 70% of Week 10's Weight

D.E. Front Squat 6x2 (30 seconds rest between sets) same weight as week 10 ***can be performed regular or to a box***

PUMP FOCUS (45 seconds rest between sets)

Bodyweight Walking Lunge 3x11 per leg

Goblet Squats 12,10,8 @ 80% of Week 10's Weight

Sissy Squats 2x10

Glute Ham Raise or Leg Curl 12,10,8 @ 80% of Week 10's Weight

Calf Raise 3x25 @ 70% of Week 10's Weight

CORE FOCUS (15-30 seconds rest between sets)

Hanging Leg Raise 2x15

McGill Curl-Up 6 reps (3/leg; Hold each rep 10 seconds)

W12D3-GW REST

W12D4-GW

STRENGTH FOCUS (2-3 minutes rest between sets)

Narrow Grip Bench Press 3x5 @ 70% of Week 10's Weight

D.E. Push Press 6x3 (45 seconds rest between sets) same weight as Week 10

Military Press 2x5 @ 70% of Week 10's Weight

PUMP FOCUS (45 seconds rest between sets)

Barbell Front Raise 12,10 @ 80% of Week 10's Weight

Dumbbell Lateral Raise 2x11 @ 80% of Week 10's Weight

Bent Over Lateral Raise 15,12,10 @ 80% of Week 10's Weight

Lying Tricep Extensions 3x11 @ 80% of Week 10's Weight

Straight Bar Tricep Cable Pushdowns 15,12 @ 80% of Week 10's Weight

Straight Bar Tricep Cable Pushdowns 1 x 30 light

CORE FOCUS (15-30 seconds rest between sets)

Ab Wheel Rollouts 3x10

W12D5-GW

STRENGTH FOCUS (2-3 minutes rest between sets)

Power Shrug 3x3 @ 70% of Week 10's Weight

Farmer's Walk 2x100ft @ 70% of Week 10's Weight

PUMP FOCUS (45 seconds rest between sets)

Double D Handle Lat Pulldown 15,12,10,20 @ 80% of Week 10's Weight

Bent Over Barbell Row 3x11 @ 80% of Week 10's Weight

Dumbbell Row 1x20 light

Barbell Cheat Curls 3x6 @ 80% of Week 10's Weight

Incline Dumbbell Curls 2x12 @ 80% of Week 10's Weight

Preacher Curls 2x15 @ Same as Week 10's Weight

Bodyweight Calf Raises 2 x max reps

No core focus today.

W12D6-GW REST

W12D7-GW REST

This concludes Week 12 of the *Bradbury Muscle Course*.

Congratulations! You have completed the full 12-week program. I am certain you have seen a visible transformation and tremendous strength gains. You should be proud of yourself! When I said this is the last program you ever need, I meant it! Now you simply go back to week 1 and repeat the program again to keep on growing. You can repeat this program for years and continue to see strength and physical improvements.

39

Movement Library

This is an overview and tips on how to perform every single movement of the *Bradbury Muscle Course*. There are many movements involved to craft a stellar physique and nobody has time for guesswork. You must master all of them and this takes precious time. This movement library's aim is to shorten your learning curve considerably. You will learn the basic techniques of the movements. You will also learn valuable tips from in the trenches to improve your performance. Please understand even the simplest of movements can take years to master. I will include a detailed how to and why for every single movement. If needed I will also include a picture demo to simplify the movement for you. There are countless ways people perform these movements. However, be rest assured if you perform them exactly as displayed in this book you will be setting yourself up to recruit maximal muscle in the safest manner possible.

CHEST

Bench Press - Wrap your thumbs around the bar. You must crush the bar with your grip. Feet firmly planted on the ground. Squeeze shoulder blades back and down by spreading your chest. Bring the bar down under control to about nipple level of your chest. Drive the bar back up to lockout. Butt must stay on bench at all times. You will use barbell or dumbbells. This is the king of upper body lifts. Use a spotter!

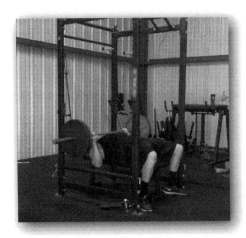 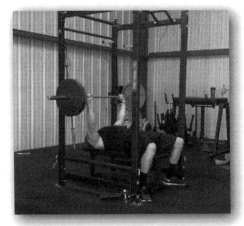

Incline Bench Press - Bench is set at an incline of 30-45 degrees, however it is wise to work all different incline angles. Wrap your thumbs around the bar. You must crush the bar with your grip. Feet firmly planted on the ground. Squeeze shoulder blades back and down by spreading your chest. Bring the bar under control to just below the collarbone. Drive the bar back up to lockout. Butt must stay on bench at all times. You will use a barbell or dumbbells. Use a spotter! This movement blasts your upper pecs and is a wonderful upper body strength builder.

Dips - Use parallel dip bars, or preferably a dip station that the bars angle out slightly to accommodate all sizes of people. Grab and squeeze bars as hard as possible. Under control lower yourself until your shoulders are at or slightly below your elbows. No half reps! Press yourself back up to start position. The further you lean forward the more chest you use. The more upright you are, the triceps will do most of the work. Use bodyweight or add weight with a dip belt. This is an awesome upper body builder!

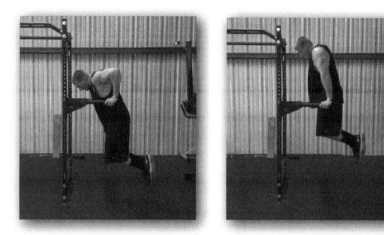

Chest Fly - Using dumbbells, band or even chains you will simply pretend you are going to hug a very large tree trunk while laying on a bench. Slowly descend your arms down and focus on getting an incredible stretch of the pecs. Once full stretch is reached, reverse the action and come up and contract the pecs forcefully at the top of the movement. Make sure to warm up into this movement with light weights as it can be demanding on your delicate shoulder structures. Focus solely on getting a maximal stretch and a maximal contraction every single rep. Do not turn this movement into a lifting contest. You will be able to use heavier and heavier weights with time, but they must always be focused reps. This move provides a great chest pump.

Narrow Grip Bench Press - This one is hard to beat for building mass in the inner chest and the triceps. Heavy weight can be used and your triceps will grow like weeds. It is the same as the bench press with a barbell, however, you will take a narrow grip with hands about 8"-14" apart. You do not want to have hands too close together as this put your wrists in danger when heavy weight is used. Use a spotter. This movement will help you stretch out your shirtsleeves in no time!

BACK

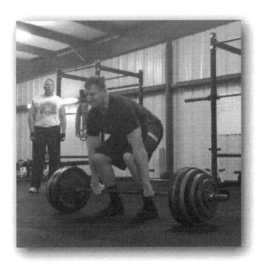 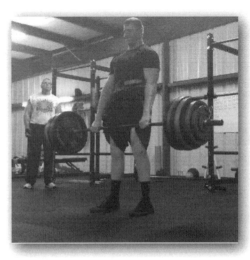

Deadlift - The honest test of full body strength and power. You cannot cheat this movement and the bar either comes up or not. Not to mention it works hundreds of muscles and is an extreme mass builder. Predominately a back exercise, but also a full body power movement. You will simply put a bar on the ground and lift it up until standing. Place your feet under your hips and the barbell very close to your shins. Bend down keeping your back in it's neutral position. Grasp the bar tightly. Some people use an alternating grip. I prefer a double over hand "hook" grip (as pictured) as this is much safer for your biceps. Brace your core, take a deep belly breath, and lift the bar by driving with legs first until standing fully erect. Start light to master proper technique. Never allow your back to round over as this can be devastating to your spinal structures. If you cannot establish a proper starting position with a neutral spine, simply put the bar up in a power rack on the pins just below knee height. This will allow a proper starting position. Then as you progress simply start each workout with the bar a touch lower and lower until it's finally on the floor. Pictured is my very first 600lb deadlift.

Power Shrug - The power shrug is a staple in our program. It builds tremendous traps and an impressive upper back. It also enhances full body explosiveness. This movement is a hidden gem and most people don't

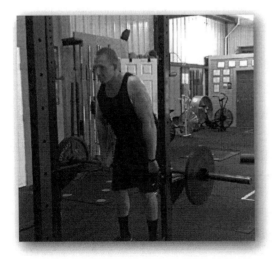 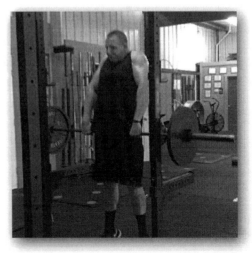

even know about it! You can use very heavy weights. You place the bar on power rack pins or rack at mid-thigh height when in starting position. You will get set by taking a deep belly breath and bracing your core tightly. Then explosively drive with your legs and shrug the weight up for a maximal contraction of the traps. Control your descent back down to starting position on the pins. Allow your traps to stretch on the eccentric (down) portion of lift. In essence, you are cheating the weight up to overload the traps and upper back and this works quite well to build slabs of muscle up there. Feel free to use wrist straps on your heavy sets. If for some odd reason you do not have a power rack or adjustable rack, you can perform this movement similar to a hang clean. Start with the weight at arms length. Then slide the bar down your thighs until the bar reaches the top of the knee. From there explosively reverse the action to perform the shrug portion.

Farmer's Walk - This is the most underrated exercise on earth! It is so simple and is incredible for increasing full body mass. You simply pick up very heavy dumbbells or farmer's walk handles loaded with weights and carry them. Make sure to use proper deadlift form for the start. Walk tall and brace your core the entire distance. This strongman staple is very fun and challenging. These will turn your grip into a jaws of life. This movement makes your whole body stronger and you'll never miss a heavy deadlift due to a weak grip again.

Shrugs - With a barbell or dumbbells you will simply shrug the weight up. Attempt to raise your shoulders up to your ears and feel your traps working. Do not raise shoulders up and then rotate them backwards. I do not know where or why people started doing that, but it is time for it to die. Simply raise shoulders up for a big squeeze at the top and then down for a good stretch every single rep. This builds your traps and upper back. it is also a great movement to improve posture.

T-Bar Row - This should also be a staple in any serious program. I prefer the old school bar in the corner or secured in a landmine. You place a double d handle on the bar up close to the sleeve on one end. You can also use a T-Bar row machine. Grab the handle and stand up. With a slight bend in the knees, bend over at the waist and keep your spine neutral the entire set. Allow the apparatus to stretch your lats and back muscles on the way down. Reverse action and come up and contract your back muscles and bring handle up to your upper abs. This is an awesome back builder!

Bent Over Barbell Row - This is another classic back builder. Great for adding mass to the entire back. Also, it gives your hamstrings a challenge. You will get a barbell and bend over with slightly bent knees. Make sure to keep spine neutral. Allow weight to stretch lats and then reverse the action and bring the bar up to anywhere between your belly button and your low chest. Go to where it feels right. Make sure to really squeeze every rep and feel back working. A pro tip: lead with your elbows to fully engage your back. Think as if your arms just connect you to the bar and you move the weight by raising your elbows.

Dumbbell Row - You can do this on a bench or on your feet. It is best to do one arm at a time. Either way it is a great way to focus on a full range of motion. Using a bench gives the lower back a break and promotes good technique. Dumbbell rows are perfect for higher reps or rep-outs to promote an incredible pump. Allow lats to stretch on the down portion. Focus on leading with your elbow to fully stimulate your back muscles. If you are using a bench, place your right hand and right knee on the bench. Then your left foot on the floor and row with your left arm. Then repeat with the other side.

Chinup/Pullup - Everyone should be able to perform pullups. Do not swing around like a spider monkey. Do these strict always. Your shoulders will thank you down the road and not to mention you'll develop an impressive back. You will go from arms straight in a hanging position to your chin over the bar utilizing full range of motion. Like dips, never do half reps. If you do things right, you will have a right conclusion. You can add weight on a dip belt when your bodyweight gets too easy. If you cannot do a single pullup as of yet do not fret. You can either use a pullup/dip assistance machine or you can utilize a band for pullups. These apparatuses will take off resistance to allow you to do your reps. Another option is to grab a workout buddy and do partner pullups. You pull as hard as you can and your partner assists just enough to help you perform a rep. This is the best way to get your first pullup. All methods will work. With the *Bradbury Muscle Course* your entire back and biceps will get exponentially stronger and pullups will become easy. Let's be clear, a chinup is when you grab the bar with an underhand grip. A pullup is when you grab the bar with an overhand grip.

Lat Pulldown - This is a movement similar to the pullup. Except you move the bar, instead of your body. You will utilize a cable and an attachment. You will use a regular lat pulldown bar or a double d handle in our program. This exercise is great for pumping up the lats and being able to focus on the muscles working. Please understand this movement does not replace pullups. It works in conjunction with pullups and vice versa. If the program calls for pullups, do pullups.

Dumbbell Pullovers - If you are under 25 years of age this movement can aid in expanding your rib cage. If you are a little older than 25 it may not have the same effect, however it is a great way to stretch the chest and build lats. Lay across a bench with shoulders on the bench. Take a single dumbbell and grip the head of the dumbbell with both hands. Allow dumbbell to stretch behind your head. You should feel a great stretch in your ribcage and chest. Then contract the lats to bring it up over your chest. You can keep arms straight or have a very slight bend in the elbows. This movement is never a bad idea to cool down with after an upper body workout for a great stretch.

Back Extensions - You will get on a back extension machine or a glute ham developer. You will place feet securely into the apparatus. Have the pads at the very top of your quads. Then lower yourself down until you are in a "L" shape and then come back up. Be careful not to over do it and hyperextend your back. You should be focusing on using your spinal erectors on every rep. This is a good movement to build up the lower back muscles, which are vital for low back health.

Reverse Hyper - You will need a reverse hyper machine. At my gym, we have a Rogue/Westside version and love it. This movement will feel awesome after heavy squats or deadlifts as it is works wonders for lower back recovery. Simply, put your feet into the strap or rollers and place the crease of your hip up to the table portion and grab the handles. You will brace your core the entire time. Raise the strap/rollers up and contract the low back and glutes. You will control it down only about a quarter of the way and then allow apparatus to swing down and swing back up into the next rep. The swing portion of the rep is actually the most beneficial as it can help to traction your spine.

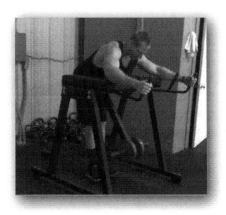 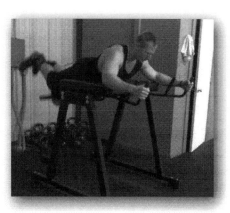

SHOULDERS

Military Press - An old school favorite. This basic movement will build impressive strength and size in the upper body. Also, it works wonders for core stabilization. Place your feet under your hips and grasp the barbell slightly wider than shoulder width apart. Crush the bar with your grip. Brace your abs and contract glutes as hard as possible to maintain a neutral spine. Avoid leaning back at all costs as this can injure low back. Press the bar straight up and over your head and then return to starting position. This movement works miracles for your overall shoulder health. It is also well known to help increase your bench press considerably.

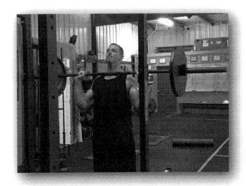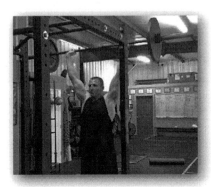

Dumbbell Shoulder Press - This movement works like the Military Press. However, you have the instability of the dumbbells and some lower back relief from the seated position. This is an incredible mass builder for the shoulders. Be seated on a bench, preferably with a back rest set at 90 degrees. Start dumbbells by the shoulder for a good stretch. Then powerfully press them up to the top.

Front Raise - You will use dumbbells or a barbell. Keep arms straight and raise them up to the front. Feel your frontal deltoid working and do these under strict control with moderate weight. Do not get reckless with these. With dumbbells you can do alternating working one arm at a time. These are great for shoulder definition and strengthening the front deltoid.

Dumbbell Lateral Raise - You can do these standing or seated. Have your arms down close to your pockets with a slight bend in the elbow. Focusing on using the side deltoid, raise the dumbbells up and away from your body out to the side for a strong contraction at the top of the movement. Then slowly return back to start position. These are awesome for increasing shoulder definition.

Dumbbell Bent Over Lateral Raise - Most programs neglect the posterior deltoid. We will not be so ignorant! We attack the posterior deltoid from many angles including direct work with this movement. I love to do this using an incline bench. You place your chest on the bench and allow arms to stretch in down position. Reverse action and come up for a strong contraction of the posterior deltoid. Make sure to tilt dumbbells at the very top just like if you were pouring out water from a cup to further engage the posterior deltoid. This muscle is vital for balanced shoulder health and upper body strength. Our program maximizes this muscle. It is a shame that many other programs do not even address it!

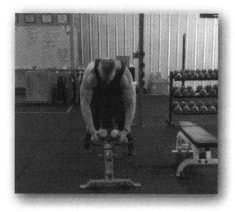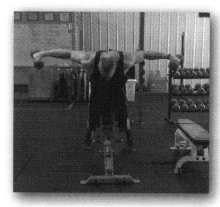

Y-T-I Complex - You also lean against an incline bench. This complex involves 3 movements. You use your arms and perform a Y shape for the allotted reps, then a T for the allotted reps and finally finish with the I for the allotted reps. If it is 1x8 per position you'll perform all 8 reps of Y's, then immediately to 8 reps of T's, and then immediately to 8 reps of I's. I like this order best since you are strongest on the I's at the very end. This is a quick way to hit all deltoids and produces a great pump.

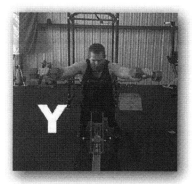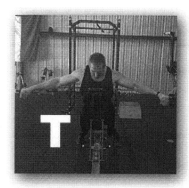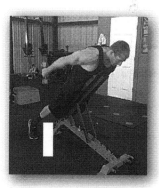

D.E. Push Press - You use a weight that is about 50-60% of your estimated 1 rep max. If your shoulder press estimated 1 rep max is 200, you can tack on 30% and you'll be fairly close to guessing your 1 rep max push press. It is estimated that for most people you can push press roughly 30% more weight than a shoulder press. Then you take 50-60% of your estimated one rep max push press and that will be the weight you use. Remember, we are more concerned with bar speed with the dynamic effort method. If you load it up and it feels heavy and slow take weight off. If you can explosively drive the bar to lockout with great speed your weight selection is on point. To perform the movement set up just like the military press. You will then brace abs and take a deep belly breath. Then dip straight down by slightly bending your knees and hips. Explode with your legs and hips to give momentum to the bar and finish by pressing hard all the way to the top. In simple terms, you will dip, drive and press.

Upright Row - This movement works your deltoids and traps extremely well. I would not suggest going super heavy on these and stick to moderate weights to achieve a crazy strong pump. Stand with bar at arms length. Put your hands about a foot apart. A wide hand placement isolates the deltoids more. Then raise bar by leading with your elbows and contract your deltoids hard. Bring bar up to about nipple level. Do not over do it by raising bar excessively high. Just come up to the point you feel your deltoids contract.

BICEPS

Barbell Cheat Curl - This is the king of bicep mass builders. The big guns in the business use this technique to pack on sheer size to their biceps. You simply do a barbell curl, but use very heavy weight. When you can no longer do the reps in a strict manner, then use your hips to hitch the weight up and give it momentum. Once you help it get a little momentum, curl with all of your might and curl the weight up. Once up, make sure to squeeze very hard and then lower slowly. This cheating method serves to blast your biceps with extreme overload. They respond by getting huge! Some people will scoff at this technique, however look at their arms and they most likely rival a 12 year olds. Cheat curls have been used for decades to build only the best arms in the game. This overload technique will help your biceps get massive.

Zottman Curls - You will use dumbbells for this movement. It literally works your entire bicep and forearm with it's unique twisting movement. You will curl the dumbbells up with hands in a palms up position. At the top, slowly rotate your hands into a palms out position and lower the weight slowly. This subtle rotation works wonders for stimulating the biceps and growing impressive forearms.

Concentration Curls - This movement is a great finisher for the biceps. It delivers a great pump. It also focuses on building the peak of the biceps. Brace yourself with your non-working arm and let the other arm dangle with the dumbbell in hand. Letting your arm hang creates a more intense pump. With extreme concentration, raise the dumbbell only by flexing the biceps. Bring the dumbbell up to the shoulder of the same arm. Finish with a strong squeeze and then lower slowly.

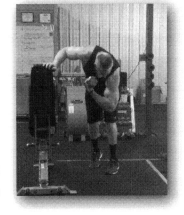

Incline Curls - This is one of my favorite bicep builders. Gives you a great stretch at the bottom of the movement. Great for adding mass to your arms. You simply sit on a 45 degree incline bench and allow arms to stretch into bottom position. Reverse the action and curl the dumbbell up for a big squeeze at the top. This movement is hard to beat for achieving an incredible pump.

Preacher Curls - These can be done with dumbbells, EZ bar, or a barbell. You can do one arm at a time if you'd like. All the world class arms have this movement in their arsenal and you should too. Gives you an awesome stretch and eliminates any cheating. You don't have to use extremely heavy weights to get the benefit of these. Rather, focus on constant tension and watch your arms blow up! Set up on a preacher bench and go down to full stretch and then up for a big squeeze.

Hammer Curls - You grab some dumbbells and curl them up with a neutral grip with palms facing each other. The brachialis and the brachioradialis are not as popular as the biceps, but play a key role in overall arm size. The hammer curl and the Zottman curl build these muscles to their maximum potential!

Reverse Curls - You can use a barbell or dumbbells. Grip with a palms down grip and crush the bar. Then you will curl up. Keep your wrist slightly extended the entire movement to further develop the top of your forearm.

Dumbbell Curl - simply perform a curl using a dumbbell. You can do them seated or standing. You can do both arms at the same time or alternating. When you "run the rack" I'd recommend curling with both arms at the same time.

TRICEPS

French Press - The triceps need to be massive to fill up your shirt sleeves. This exercise is perfect for packing on size to every part of your triceps. You take an EZ bar or a dumbbell and put it over your head. Keeping elbows in tight close to your ears, slowly lower until you feel a good stretch along the back of your arms. Then reverse and come up for a big squeeze at the very top. Always warm up well on any triceps movement as the elbows can get aggravated quite easily. You can also do one arm at a time with a single dumbbell.

Triceps Cable Pushdown - This one can be used with a straight bar, V-handle, or a rope. Excellent for pumping the triceps up like a balloon. If you don't have a cable apparatus, you can always use a band to perform movement. You get a good stretch in the up position and then pushdown trying to isolate the triceps. Make sure to get a strong contraction at the bottom of the movement with a slight pause. Keep your elbows glued to your sides the entire set.

Narrow Grip Bench Press - This one is hard to beat for building mass in the inner chest and the triceps. Heavy weight can be used and your triceps will grow like weeds. It is the same as the bench press with a barbell, however, you will take a narrow grip with hands about 8"-14" apart. You do not want to have hands too close together as this put your wrists in danger when very heavy weight is used. Use a spotter. This movement will help you stretch out your shirtsleeves in no time!

Lying Tricep Extensions - These are also known as "skullcrushers." You will lay down on a bench and you can use a barbell, EZ bar, or dumbbells. Bring the bar down slowly to your forehead (dumbbells to the ears). Then extend elbows to lockout. Do not get reckless and turn this into an actual skullcrusher! Be sure to use a light enough weight to feel your muscles working. The elbows are delicate so start by warming them up with very light weight. This is one of the best movements for mass. Make sure to have a spotter.

Dumbbell Kickbacks - This is a finisher movement and it will pump your triceps up like crazy. Bend over at the waist with a flat back. Glue your elbows to your sides. Using only your triceps, extend the elbows until your arms are straight and triceps are fully contracted. Then lower slowly and repeat. Many people drop their elbows when they get tired, don't do this! You can also do one arm at a time, by putting the non-working side's arm and leg on a bench.

Incline Single Arm French Press - You will simply do a french press leaning against an incline bench. Do not sit as the dumbbell will hit the top of the seat. Just lean against the incline. Make sure the incline bench you have won't tip over before doing your set. The incline gives you an incredible stretch and you will definitely feel the difference.

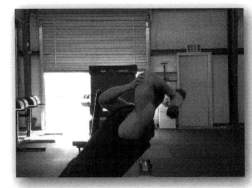

Bench Dips - Put your palms on the edge of a bench or plyometrics box. Then put your feet up on another bench or box. You can add resistance by putting plates in your lap. You dip down by bending elbows and then reverse action and come back up. You will get intense contractions in the triceps during this movement. I love this movement for triceps definition.

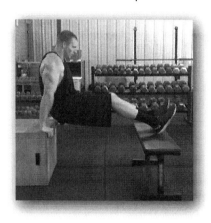

LEGS

Back Squat - If I could only do one exercise the rest of my life it would be the squat. This is best for building full body power and size. Squats will give you an incredible natural boost of muscle building hormones. If you increase your squat your whole body will grow more muscle. You can place the bar on your traps in a high bar position or you can put the bar just below the spine of the scapula in a low bar position. It's your call here. Personally, I use a high bar position until the final phase of 5x5 and I switch it to the low bar position. You will put your feet slightly wider than shoulder width apart and point toes out slightly. Make sure your heels stay glued to the floor the entire set. To start decent, shove your hips back and down. Then bend at the knees. You will go down under control until your hip crease is just below the top of your knee. Then you drive into the bar back up to start position. Make sure to hold onto the bar with your hands. A thumbless grip is acceptable when using a low bar position. Do not violently bounce out of the bottom. Keep your spine neutral the entire set. Brace your core and take a deep belly breath before descending. Maintain tightness the entire set. It is a great idea to have a qualified trainer teach you how to squat correctly.

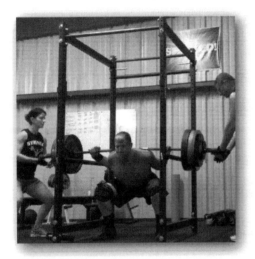 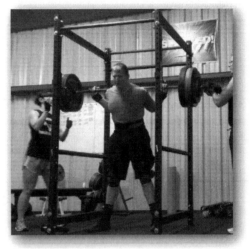

Front Squat - The front squat is similar to the back squat, however the bar is on your shoulders on the front side of your body. You can leave your fingertips on the bar with it resting on your shoulders with elbows pointed straight ahead. This is called the "rack position." You can also cross your arms and point elbows straight ahead. Whatever you do make sure your elbows stay up as high as possible and point them at the wall in front of you. This is a quad-dominant exercise and must be executed with the torso very erect. If you have trouble with this movement do goblet squats until you gain the flexibility needed to squat with an upright torso. The concepts are the same as the back squat, however, your knees will go out further over your toes. This is to help keep torso erect. Just make sure to keep heels down and reach depth.

Lunges - This can be done with bodyweight, dumbbells or barbell on your back. These build serious mass on your legs. You want to take a large step, then lower slowly until your knee is about 1" off of the ground and then stand. I prefer to do walking lunges. Do not allow your front knee to travel too far out over your toes as this can aggravate your knees.

Belt Squat - This is a great way to pump your legs, gain flexibility for squatting and it doesn't compress your spine. You simply set up two small boxes or stack plates. Grab a dip belt and put weight on it. Stand on the boxes and squat down. You can really squat deep with this method. Make sure to go at a smooth pace to maintain balance. Work to maintain proper squat mechanics. This is a great way to increase training volume to build muscle without being too hard on your back.

D.E. Back Squat - Dynamic effort method uses a lighter load usually around 50-60% of your 1RM with little rest in between sets. You focus on moving the bar as fast as possible. You can do the D.E. Squat to a box if you so choose or free standing. You can also add chains or bands to accommodate resistance. Make sure to account for chain weight or band tension with your load. You can also just use the bar with weights. Simply descend under control and once you reach bottom you will explode up. Your mission is to move the bar as fast as possible from the bottom up. If it ever feels slow or heavy, lower the weight.

Goblet Squat - Grab a kettlebell or a dumbbell and hold it very close to your chest. Put your elbows down the side of the KB/DB. Then using proper squat mechanics, squat down until your elbows are near the inside of your knees and then rise. Keep your chest up the whole time. This is a fool-proof way to learn how to squat correctly.

Glute Ham Raise - You will need a glute ham developer machine (GHD machine). You put your feet into the pads with the foot plate. Have the other pads at mid-upper quad level. The start position is like the beginning of a back raise. Your legs are straight and you are bent over with your head down by the floor. Perform a back raise and then pull with your hamstrings and curl your legs. Most people find they cannot perform even a single rep at first without help. Curl your legs and then fire your glutes to bring your hip through. Then slowly lower back to start position. This is a relatively unknown movement that is a staple in any serious strength program. It will make your squat and deadlift go up exponentially. It targets most people's weakness, the posterior chain.

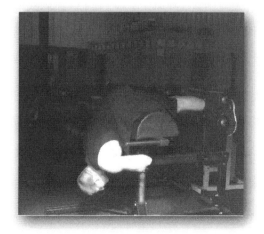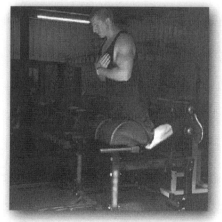

Sissy Squat - Don't let the name fool you, this is a quad killer. I really consider it a natural leg extension. You will do these free standing. Grab ahold of something for balance. You can place a 2-4" sturdy block under heels or just stay on your toes. Put your feet about hip width. Keeping your body completely straight from neck to knees, go up on your toes and bend at the knees and go down. You will have to lean back while performing the move. Then reverse the action back up to start position. This is a great isolation exercise for the quads. It will give you great definition. In our program, we use it for higher volume so you don't need to add weight. I wouldn't recommend trying to use a bunch of weight on this exercise. Stay in control and stop immediately if it bothers your knees. You can substitute bodyweight squats if you cannot do sissy squats.

Bulgarian Split Squat - This is a great unilateral movement that promotes muscular balance. You put your trailing (non-working side) foot up on a bench. Then step out similar to a lunge position. Then slowly lower yourself until trailing knee is close to the ground. Once you master technique you can add weight with dumbbells. This is another great way to maximize leg development.

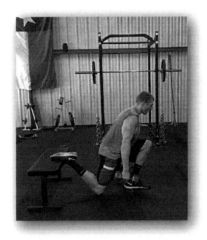

Romanian Deadlift - A great movement to develop hamstring strength and flexibility. It also works to build your low back muscles. You'll take a barbell and have a very slight bend in your knees. Keeping your spine in a neutral position, you'll descend the bar down in front of you towards your toes. You will strongly feel your hamstrings stretch. When you feel a good stretch then return back up to the starting position.

Leg Press - Find a leg press machine and follow manufacturer's directions closely. Do not allow apparatus to come down too far and round lower back on the seat as this can cause an injury.

Leg Curl - Find a leg curl machine and follow manufacturer's directions closely.

Calf Raises - I like to use a 2"x4" and a dip belt with plates on it. Simply get a good stretch on the calves and then raise all the way up onto your toes. Focus on a strong contraction at the top! You can also use a calf machine if you have access to one.

CORE

Ab Wheel Rollouts - This is one of the best dynamic core movements you can do. Maintaining stabilization throughout a range of motion is one of the key roles the abs play. The ab wheel is exceptional for training the abs for maximal stabilization and bracing while performing a movement. Keep your spine neutral at all times. Do not let your back "sway" at all as this causes lots of compression on your delicate spinal structures. Keeping your midline stable, rollout as far as you can without losing midline stabilization and return. You can buy an ab wheel for a few bucks at a sporting goods store or you can also use a barbell with plates on it.

McGill Curl Up - This is a very subtle exercise. You must work hard and contract forcefully. It really shouldn't appear that you are doing much movement. You'll lay down and put your hands under your low back. Bend one knee to 90 degrees and keep the other leg straight on the ground. Then contract the abs forcefully and feel your upper back, shoulders and head become unweighted off of the ground. Keep chin tucked and hold maximal contraction for 10 seconds. This is an awesome spine saving core movement. It also teaches you how to brace your core and generate stabilization.

Hanging Leg Raise - You can use a pair of ab straps or do them by simply hanging from a chinning bar. Make sure to really focus and feel abs working the entire range of motion and do not turn this into a swinging contest. Raise knees up to chest and feel abs contract and then lower and repeat.

Turkish Get Up - See Turkish Get Up chapter for detailed instruction.

Plank / Side Plank - Keep body rigid and straight at all times. Do not push your butt high into the air or sway your lower back. Stay straight as a board. This is a simple, yet extremely effective exercise to promote midline stability and low back health.

Can I use olympic lifts in the *Bradbury Muscle Course*?

Yes. Feel free to substitute olympic lifts or variations in for the power shrug. However, please understand that while olympic lifts are entertaining and can build power, they are not the best option for muscle mass development. The power shrug also builds tremendous power and develops loads of muscle. You could substitute power cleans for power shrugs for an entire 12-week cycle to spice things up.

Is the *Bradbury Muscle Course* good for sports?

In most sports, bigger and stronger muscles presents the athlete with an unfair advantage to their peers. Yes, this is a superb program for sports that benefit from increased muscle mass and strength. Not to mention, better flexibility and improved joint integrity thanks to proper resistance training. I would recommend that you make sure that sport-specific drills and conditioning are being trained in conjunction with the Bradbury Muscle Course. Often, sport practice, scrimmages and even games serves this purpose the best. I have never really bought into the idea that you should attempt to mimic your sport in the weight room by doing weight training movements that are eerily similar to the sport being played. The fact is the game is played on the field or court. Practice your sport there with sport-specific drills and playing the actual sport. Do not do synchronized dumbbell dances that look like your sport. Remember, bigger and stronger athletes win and win big in most sports. You have two running backs... one squats 650 and the other squats 135... you are on the 2 yard line and it's 4th & goal.... who are you giving the ball to? Do the basics and do them better than your competition if you want to win.

I have a physical ailment that won't allow me to do <insert any exercise> what should I do instead?

Everyone is different and some movements do not work for some people who have past injuries and/or other ailments. This is okay and no worries you can still benefit greatly from the Bradbury Muscle Course. The answer to this question is understanding the concept. Understand the concept of the intended exercise and replace original movement with a movement you can perform without trouble. Example, you can't do lying tricep extensions, but you can do cable pushdowns with no problem. Just sub the cable pushdown for the lying tricep extensions. Your triceps will still get stimulation and grow.

I don't have the right equipment to do <insert any exercise>?

Find a way or make a way. Join a legit gym that will allow to perform all of the movements. If you are a garage dude you'll have to improvise or buy/build equipment that will work for you. This is one major disadvantage to training in a garage. However, you can still make awesome gains by improvising. This program is designed for simplicity and most of it can be performed with minimal equipment. You can sub the cable pushdowns with a good set of bands. Be creative.

Can I add <insert any program> concepts to the *Bradbury Muscle Course*?

No. Do the program as it is intended or don't do it at all. If something works why be foolish and try to tinker with it?

My half-cousin Bobby said that lifting weights is dangerous, is that true?

Listen. Whenever you strive towards any new endeavor you will have naysayers. It doesn't matter what you are doing they will come out and try to belittle or discourage you. This is out of nothing but fear that you'll show up at the next family event jacked as hell. Always be kind, but you don't need to listen to people like that. Prove to them that they are goofballs when you become extremely muscular and shredded to bits. Then you tell ol' Bobby that he was exactly right because after you started lifting weights you got all swole up.

Can women do the *Bradbury Muscle Course* or will they get too bulky?

Let's debunk this goofy myth right now. The best way to shed fat and transform your body is through resistance training and proper diet. It is insanely common for people to think that women if they lift heavy weights will magically turn into the hulk and look dreadfully "MANLY." However, the opposite is true. Truly, 99.9% of women who join a gym or hire a trainer are desperately wanting to get a "leaner and toner look." Trust me I know. However, many slave away on a cardio machine, sweating buckets and never get the results they want. Women will get unbelievable results and look incredibly lean with great muscle tone if they'd just hit the weights! More precisely, the Bradbury Muscle Course is optimal for women to do just that. The only way for a woman to get bulky lifting weights is: 1) use illegal anabolic steroids 2) eat way too much food. Avoid those two things and you will develop a stunning physique. Ladies, truly if you want to own the beach get your diet dialed in and do this program and watch the magic happen!

What can I substitute for sissy squats?

Many people find that at first sissy squats may be uncomfortable. I used to have issues with "jumper's knee" and have found sissy squats have really helped to strengthen my quads and my knee pain is gone. The key is to start by just going down a little and going slowly. Do not move too fast or go down too far as this can agitate your knee(s). You can also place a barbell in a rack and hang onto the bar against the rack and relieve some resistance when starting out. As you get more and more comfortable with the movement then you can do them freestanding or by hanging on with one arm against the rack for balance. They will get easier as your quads get stronger so hang in there. Aim to work up to 50 reps in a row freestanding and you will be a master of sissy squats. However, if you have knee issues and cannot do sissy squats, it is okay! You can simply substitute them with bodyweight squats and get a similar adaptation.

How can I reduce soreness?

First get your diet dialed in and make sure you are eating plenty of protein. Second get your supplement regimen going. Third give yourself time. This program is designed to shock your muscles periodically throughout the program. If you've never lifted before you will be very sore, but stick it out! Your body will adapt and soreness will be less intense. Truly, you will never not be sore, but it won't ever be as bad as the first few weeks.

Why did you write this book?

Honestly, I was motivated by the people who really wanted to get results, but never got them. It become glaringly apparent that so many people were confused. They really wanted a lean, muscular physique, but were going after it in a completely incorrect manner. It truly was a sign of mass confusion. I wanted to give you a results-based blueprint on exactly how to build muscle and how to get lean to show off your new muscles. To me, 99% of people join a gym or something because they want to look and feel good. Sadly, because of sheer misunderstanding, people who were either taught or believed what they thought would work, just does not work. I wanted to create a program that any man or woman on the face of the earth could utilize and finally get the jaw-dropping results they so deeply desired. This book is the solution. If you follow every simple step and do the program you will develop an incredible physique. That is the exact reason why I wrote this book.

How many times should you go through the entire 12-week program?

If you want to keep growing... keep going.

I feel really good can I go hard on an assigned growth week?

Accumulated fatigue is a filthy animal. CNS fatigue is even filthier. More is not better. Have you ever known someone who talk about how they "work out" for hours everyday and have no results? I know I have! Don't be foolish and trust me. Follow the program, if it is a growth week do the growth week correctly. It will pay huge dividends down the road.

What if I cannot do a single bodyweight pullup or dip?

You can easily get assistance to perform reps. You can add a high quality band or use a gravitron-type machine, if available, to help out by taking some resistance off. A workout partner can push you up. I really prefer that you do real pull-ups versus always using the lat pulldown. You will be shocked at how quickly you will get your first pullup and dip with this program. It is a great idea to work a few negatives with your bodyweight to build strength and confidence. A negative is simply jumping up with your chin over the bar and then lowering yourself as slowly as possible. You can also do negatives with dips.

How do I estimate my 1 rep max?

weight x reps x 0.0333 + weight = estimated 1 rep max

Example:

225# x 8 reps x 0.0333 + 225# = 284.94 is estimated 1 rep max

Please understand that this is an estimated 1 rep max based on a formula and calculations. Generally, this common formula is quick to use and gives you a fairly accurate estimate. However, to know your real 1 rep max you should perform a 1 rep max test.

Can I use bands/chains in with the Bradbury Muscle Course?

Absolutely! I prefer chains as they have a more natural feel and are less demanding on your body. To mix it up, you could do the entire 12-weeks using chains on bench or squat. This will give it a different feel and shock your muscles into further growth. Be sure to only do this periodically and for the most part perform the Bradbury Muscle Course exactly how it is written. Also, be careful not to get too overzealous with accommodating resistance as it can lead to overtraining.

On max out week 11 should I do a 1, 3, or 5 rep max?

You get to choose whichever you prefer. 1 rep max's can be quite demanding for some people, however you will learn your true 1 rep max. If you don't like the idea of doing a max single, go with a 3 or 5 rep max. Either way, you can track strength gains every time you go through the 12 week cycle. Another good idea, is to do a 5 rep max on squat, 3 rep max on bench, and a 1 rep max on deadlift. You can shuffle those around the next time through by switching the numbers around with the exercises. This way you will have an accurate 1 rep max test result on the squat, bench, and deadlift every 36 weeks. You can have this without having to worry about having 3 different 1 rep max tests the same week.

Beau Bradbury CSCS, CPT is a fitness professional and facility owner in Weatherford, Texas. He is the author of the book *Bradbury Muscle Course* and has published numerous internet articles. He first started helping people change their bodies for the better at age 17. He graduated from Texas Tech University in 2011 with a Bachelor of Science in exercise science and a minor in nutrition. He is certified by the National Strength & Conditioning Association as a CSCS and the American Council on Exercise as a CPT. He passionately helps people everyday radically improve their physiques by working with them in person or through his publications.

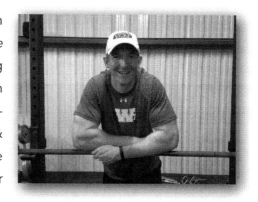

60054441R00082

Made in the USA
Middletown, DE
26 December 2017